THE PERFECT ATHLETE
WINNING WITH NUTRITION

OLIVIER DOLEUZE

CONTENTS

Introduction   v

PART ONE
NEED TO KNOW BASIS

1. Introduction to Nutrition   3
2. The Science of Nutrition   12
3. Nutrition History   24

PART TWO
BODY OF WORK

4. Physique   33
5. Muscle Function   44
6. Mental Health and Competitive Sports   57

PART THREE
BEGINNERS

7. How You Eat   71
8. Eating Fit   82
9. Getting Active   92

PART FOUR
INTERMEDIATE

10. Cooking Smart   105
11. Working Out   119

PART FIVE
EXPERIENCED

12. Fueling the Machine   131
13. Training   150

Final Words   155
Free Bonus Guide   157
References   159

© Copyright 2022 - All rights reserved.

It is not legal to reproduce, duplicate, or transmit any part of this document in either electronic means or in printed format. Recording of this publication is strictly prohibited and any storage of this document is not allowed unless with written permission from the publisher except for the use of brief quotations in a book review.

INTRODUCTION

What do you need to light a fire? You require a match or a lighter, some lighter fluid or accelerant. You'll need tinder, twigs, paper, or anything that will quickly catch flame. Oh, and of course, wood. You know the ingredients, and mostly how it all works—enough to eventually get the job done.

But you want a better fire. You want to know how to make it last longer, burn hotter, catch more efficiently. To do so, you need to learn more about how fire is made. You need to understand oxygen consumption and moisture and other factors that affect it. You need to learn which type of wood burns better and where to acquire it.

This is a pretty straightforward analogy for food, but the fire in this case is your athleticism and your performance in your sport. It's a lot more than just 'food in' equals function.

You may have all but mastered your sport and passion, but you cannot seem to make significant gains towards the next level of performance. There seems to be something missing from the equation. Pushing your body works, and you train hard. But there are times when you lag instead of surging ahead when the pressure is on. Some days you just can't seem to get enough energy. In your off-season training time you aren't making the progress you want for the next competition or event. You grab your usual snack to think about it, and analyze it. Really look at it. What are you eating?

The problem is likely your fuel. You get hungry. You eat. But is it at the right time? Is it enough to fill you up? More importantly, the question you really need to ask yourself—is this the right food? Lastly, what do I want this food to do for me?

There is no one-size-fits-all program or recipe that will magically fix your diet, perfect your eating discipline, or suddenly make you more powerful. The process is just that, a progression and a development of your knowledge about not only nutrients and dietary necessities, but most importantly, your body and exactly what it needs to become a finely tuned machine.

With in-depth studies, a closer look at why foods work the way they do, and what our bodies do with those foods, you will be able to start changing your eating habits. You will track your intake and how it affects you. Not only that, but you will see what you may have been doing wrong and be able to fix the issue. Hopefully, you will also get inspired to achieve even greater objectives as you gain the missing piece of the puzzle to complete your athletic masterpiece.

As a professional jockey, I saw dramatic changes in myself as I grew in my sport over a lifetime. Nutrition always played a vital role in my training over the course of three decades, a span of years that was also the most critical time in Sports Nutrition advancement and discovery. As nutritional knowledge grew, so did the changes in athletic expectation and the food needs of those demands. You could argue that my wins on the track were only possible due to my interest in fueling my athletic performance with the best sources of sustenance I could find. Now that I am retired and look at those trophies and achievements, I want to see others reach their own finish lines. To do that, I must share my passion for the impetus behind athletic endeavors and success.

At the end of the race, we truly are what we eat, to use the old phrase. In order to be better, we have to eat better. To be the best, you need to eat like a champion.

You have the prowess and the skills to reach every one of your goals. Now, it's time you use your formidable sporting determination to learn the methods needed to feed those ambitions and the mighty body that makes it all possible.

The first step? It all starts at the bottom with a foundation of information and understanding all of the intricate interplays of the moving parts of the system. You have the tool kit, you just need to know what each tool is for, how it's made, and when and how to use it.

PART ONE
NEED TO KNOW BASIS

CHAPTER 1
INTRODUCTION TO NUTRITION

As with any workout, it's always best to start with a bit of a warm-up! Getting the blood flowing in your veins and preparing your muscles for the work ahead is a must to make sure you don't strain anything. The same goes for your brain. Warming up to the material in this book starts with the basics. This chapter will loosen you up with some vital, foundational information and prime you for action, just like a few minutes of good old fashioned body-weight squats.

For that matter, get on your feet and do a few sets while you read!

NUTRITION

Nutrition, in the simplest scientific terms, is *how organisms consume organic substances to survive.* (Wikipedia Contributors 2019) We all know this as eating food, of course! Your rumbling stomach tells you all you need to know about when you need to feed yourself.

Today, we more commonly understand nutrition as the study of nutrients in the food we eat and how those nutrients affect and sustain the body. This study also incorporates the interplay of overall health, diseases, diet, and general wellness. Additionally, this includes the relationship of nutrition to fitness and exercise, which is the real point of this book!

Before we delve into the intricacies of how amino acid chains fuel the growth of muscles or even how carbohydrates and sugars give you energy to do those sports you love, we need to examine all of the terminology of nutrition, definitions, and meanings we will be using to perfect your athletic performance and physical health.

Grab a healthy snack and let's get to work!

TERMINOLOGY

Nutrients– To put it plainly, this word encompasses all of the substances we consume to live. This includes the macronutrients such as proteins, fats, or carbohydrates, as well as micronutrients like minerals and vitamins that we gain from both foods and supplementary additives to our diet. (Wikipedia Contributors 2019) Most people have a vague understanding of nutrients as the 'good things' we get from foods. This isn't entirely wrong as nutritional science is understood by and large, especially for the sporting individual just trying to figure out what they need to eat to be their very best!

Diet– No, we don't mean the rigorous routine of cutting out junk food you tried last spring to work on your beach body! Your diet is essentially the list of everything you eat—good and bad. Our goal here is to perfect that diet by changing the foods that it's made up of, and hone your knowledge of what your body needs to perform and to grow, or shrink, accordingly!

Calories– This one is a little tricky, mostly because of pop-culture trends and media. Everyone knows that we 'burn calories' throughout the day, and that all food has calories. These mysterious units add up to a number that either makes you gain or lose weight. Or something like that, right?

To clarify, calories, also called food calories or kcal, are units used in several sciences to define energy values. (Wikipedia Contributors 2019a) Where food is concerned, this really just gives us a baseline for understanding and measuring quantities of energy per weight of the types of food we eat and how that relates to how fast we burn, or use, that food energy.

Fortunately, in terms of fitness and exercise, the rule of simple maths does still apply. If you burn more calories than you eat, you lose body mass. If you eat more calories than you burn, you gain body mass. The trick when gaining or losing is to make sure you are eating the right kinds of calories to feed the type of mass you want to modify!

Metabolism– Metabolism encompasses all of the chemical reactions that occur within your body that convert the energy in food into usable cell energy. The cells within your body *metabolize,* or break the chemicals in food down in different ways and use the elements as building blocks for sustenance, growth, and recovery. (Wikipedia Contributors 2019b) Don't worry, that's about as complex as we will get into the microbiological workings of your body. Our purpose is to help you master your diet crafting, not make you memorize the steps of cell mitosis!

In nutritional science the term *metabolism* will often be used to describe the rate at which a person's body performs all of these processes. You have undoubtedly heard people talk about slower and faster metabolisms in regards to weight loss and gain. The same can be said about certain food groups in how quickly they can be digested and their influence on increasing your metabolic efficiency. Great foods can help program your body just as effectively as doing squats strengthens your quads.

Finally, this word can also be used to define the entire process of eating, digestion, and excretion.

Physical fitness– From our school days we all became familiar with physical activity and fitness to some degree. Physical fitness outside of PE class, however, is your overall state of well being and health.

The description or evaluation of your fitness level can also incorporate your capacity to compete in sporting events, complete physical tasks and activities, and define the ease of physicality in your daily life. The functionality and efficiency of how well your body works ties in closely with your response times, in other words, the mind-muscle connection and reflexive reaction. Another gauge is how effectively you can execute the tasks you demand of your body, or coordination. Reaction and coordination are almost impossible to separate. Training inherently develops both.

There are four general types of fitness associated with our bodies and abilities: endurance, balance, strength or power, and flexibility. Endurance defines how long our body can withstand and maintain a workload, while balance deals in muscular control and that mind-muscle connection. Strength indicates how much power we can generate from our muscles and flexibility comes from the pliability and elasticity of both our muscles, joints, ligaments, and tendons. As we explore various sports later in this book we will analyze how these fitness aspects play out in varying degrees in the different sports, and of course, how you should eat to accommodate the demands of each. (Wikipedia Contributors 2019c)

. . .

Weight management– Weight management is the act of controlling and regulating your body's ratio of fat and muscle. Some of this is based on our desires for our appearance, some on body type, and activity capacity. Moreover, weight management is affected by all of the other topics we've mentioned thus far. Your diet, activity level, and injuries or other conditional effects on your body all factor into maintaining or altering your body mass ratio and weight. It is extremely important to determine what a healthy weight and body mass ratio looks like for your body.

Dieting– In this case we mean the action not the list! The act of dieting can be any purposeful change in your diet to reach a goal, typically for a limited period of time. Dieting can also be a prescribed periodic system designed to control what you are eating for specific results. This incorporates adopting broad stroke type diets like vegetarian, vegan, carnivore, etc. Then there are more specific styled diets like *keto* and *paleo* which you may have heard of in recent years. Both have become very popular. Be very cautious when approaching these diet plans as there tends to be a lot of misinformation and misconceptions about proper implementation of them. Be sure and research a diet plan before attempting it to really find out if it suits your needs and provides sufficient nutrition for you.

Fad diets have always been a part of the amateur fitness realm and should be carefully navigated and studied before attempting them. Trends such as *carb cutting*, or any pill or product that promises drastic and quick results should be viewed with skepticism. (Fitzgerald 2004) Almost every one of these is not good for you, or they simply don't work.

If you are unsure, a registered dietitian nutritionist (RDN) can help you ascertain if a plan is right for you and how to safely apply it.

• • •

Supplements– Supplements can mean anything from vitamins and minerals to powdered protein or even adding apple cider vinegar to your diet to help balance your stomach's pH levels. Supplements are generally modified or concentrated parts of macro or micro nutrients designed to increase your intake of a specific chemical to augment a deficiency or create an abundance for growth or healing. This can include steroidal enhancers, both the actual steroids themselves and dietary supplements that encourage hormonal steroid production in the body. Of course it goes without saying that using any kind of these supplements should only ever be done with the controlled supervision of your personal medical professional.

Many products get hyper specific in the chemicals offered for very particular designs and gains. Your local vitamin shop is full of them. They are not all intrinsically bad, but be wary of what other chemicals they may contain that can be hard on your kidneys and liver as well as high levels of sugar and caffeine. Consider that you may just need to eat better or tweak your diet to accommodate your needs instead of immediately turning to these products for results.

ATHLETICISM AND SPORTS NUTRITION

Applying all of this nutritional knowledge can be of great use for any person looking to improve their health, but none so much as the person who trains to compete in amateur sporting events. Of course this holds the most importance for professional athletes. Refining what you give your body is the most integral part of creating a truly athletic physique and achieving the highest goals in your mastery of the skills in your sport.

• • •

Fuel– Putting the wrong kind of fuel in your car can cause minor damage, poor performance, or at the worst, destroy your engine. The same is true of your body. It is a machine of many interconnecting systems and engines that need the right fuel to function. Fine tuning this intake can only make it run better and last longer.

Hydration– Water comprises 60% of the human body. This should be an indicator of just how important drinking water really is, especially for athletes who exert themselves regularly and sweat intensely. This is all water use and water loss. That water has to be replaced! We all know how it feels to sweat buckets on a hot day, more so if you are working hard.

Putting it frankly, water is more important than food. Humans die more quickly from water deprivation than starvation. Not only do we need the water to sustain our organ functionality, it is crucial in the digestion of food and processing of energy as well as growth and replenishing our supplies of blood and tissue.

On top of that, water acts as our primary source of temperature regulation, thus the sweating. If that wasn't enough to drive this fact home, our brains are 73% water! So you can see why water is the most important thing we can put in our bodies. Making sure you get enough of it is not only paramount to your survival, but crucial to your success. On average, it is recommended that we drink at least two liters (64oz.) of water per day. (Water Science School 2019) This requirement only goes up the more workload you put on your system!

RECOVERY AND GROWTH

As important as it is to give the body energy to work, after the work is done we need those precious nutrient building blocks to repair damage, build more muscle, and retain the elements of our body at peak performance. You could almost argue that eating after you work out is even more important than eating before, but don't get carried away! Making sure you eat the correct amounts and types of food for all of your needs is imperative.

DIETITIANS AND NUTRITIONISTS

As mentioned above, researching for yourself is highly recommended to evaluate and understand your dietary needs. Conferring with your peers can also be a great source of advice as well as support and accountability for staying healthy.

Not to mention that this book is a great tool for moving in the right direction!

Ultimately, the best course of action for professional results is simply to consult a professional. In the pursuit of guidance and creating the perfect diet, there are many experts on the subject who you can seek out for assistance.

A local nutritionist can give you a multitude of advice and answer many questions you might have about supplements and dieting. However, most nutritionists in food industries and food sciences are primarily self taught and uncertified as dietitians. Not to say they don't know an ample amount of useful knowledge.

If you want to meet with a licensed professional, you can find registered dietitian nutritionists through your public and private medical health care providers and in many educational forums. These individuals must maintain their university-studied certification through ongoing education and have extensive scientific and health care experience to not only direct you, but also help you discover and solve food-related issues such as allergies. (Newman 2020)

. . .

Next we will get a little more intense as we explore in-depth the definitions and science of individual nutrients and where they are found and how they work. Each of these nutrients has something to offer as they compete for a dominant spot in your dietary lineup. Which one will take first place may surprise you as we begin to combine our nutritional know-how with our powerful performance prerequisites.

If you find yourself losing focus, make sure you do some jumping jacks between chapters and grab a snack for a kick of energy!

CHAPTER 2
THE SCIENCE OF NUTRITION

After you get warmed up, the next step is putting together a game plan or preparing a regimen. Knowing all of the options available and choosing the best and most effective exercise is the only way to guarantee a good workout. What muscle groups will you hit today? What do you need to work on to reach your goals? Don't waste a minute wondering what to do next.

The same goes for meals. Knowing the ins and outs of the foods you will use to fuel your gains and recovery will help you establish a winning regimen of nutrition to match your training program.

THE BREAKDOWN

For many of you, some of this information will be familiar, but getting to know the finer points of what makes up the foods we need to live and compete and how our bodies take advantage of them will become more and more important as we progress toward becoming perfect athletes. Just like the links in amino acid chains that build muscle fiber, learning the inner workings of nutrition will build a solid path forward in your athletic journey.

Nutrition science studies the effects of everything we consume and how we use these compounds to perform all of our bodily functions. The machine of the human body is an extremely intricate and complicated interplay of codependent systems. Fortunately for us, aside from diseases, abnormalities, or injuries, the majority of this machine runs autonomously as long as we feed it! The foundations of nutrition science start with the fundamentals of biology and chemistry, with a healthy dose of physics and mathematics. We can explore a bit more of the numbers and the physical activity once we have paved the groundwork of ingredients involved in driving us. ("Nutritional Science" 2021)

MACRONUTRIENTS

Macronutrients are essentially the consumable substances that humans need an abundance of to survive. Previously, methods of conveying these types of nutrients have been presented in simple charts and graphs taught to us at an early age as a pyramid or in groups of similar seeming foods. We have all heard of the *basic food groups* in some form or another, although what that means varies greatly depending on where you live and sometimes changes based on cultural interpretation. Despite some of this ambiguity, these food groups are not entirely wrong in their assignment.

Separating foods into groups like vegetables, fruits, grains and starches, meats, and so on is beneficial for simplistic understanding of nutrition, but there are many faults in this method. For example, vegetables are not actually a type of nutrient! The carbohydrates and proteins in the vegetables are what your body actually uses as nutrients. So when categorizing foods, it may come as a surprise that some vegetables fall in with complex grains, and many plants like nuts are grouped closer to meats due to their high protein content.

Of course, it is all a little more complicated, especially as you begin to cook, bake, and combine ingredients. For this reason, standardized charts have been universally added to millions of products worldwide to display the *nutritional values* in products. While the labels should not be your bible for all nutritional information, this baseline is certainly a useful and wonderful tool to assist you in choosing your meals.

PROTEINS

Since this book is predominantly for athletes and aspiring fitness enthusiasts, we have to talk about protein before any other nutrient! As an athlete you likely eat an absurd amount of this nutrient, and with good cause. You need it. Protein equals muscle, and muscles equal your strength and movement.

Proteins are long chains of organic compounds called amino acids that have specific structures which perform specific tasks, to put it as straightforwardly as possible. Proteins are the reason you can digest foods. They catalyze metabolic reactions, give your cells the ability to signal and interpret stimuli like how you know when something is hot, and they even create the foundations for replicating your DNA! Proteins are very useful molecules.

There are a total of 20 types of amino acids that our bodies regularly deal with. You don't need to know most of them unless you are really interested in enzymatic microbiology and designing your own brand of supplements, or you are a beer brewing enthusiast. Proteins are also instrumental in making beer.

While those proteins are fun and pretty handy, they aren't nearly as important as the kind we eat for sustenance. *Essential amino acids* are proteins that we cannot synthesize on our own and must be eaten in our diet, so for our purposes, this is the main type of protein we will address. (Wikipedia Contributors 2019d)

To get these proteins we literally have to add them to our bodies by consuming things that have protein in them. That way our body can take that material, break it down, and use it to maintain muscle fiber and other tissues. As we exercise, we create the demand for our body to provide more strength and ability to meet the rising workload, which then demands more materials to work with.

Foods with high concentrations of protein include the more obvious meats and poultry, but there are so many other foods that offer not only a source of protein, but also supply essential micronutrients as well as sugars and fats.

Animal protein– Beef, pork and other meats, poultry, and fish are referred to as *animal proteins*. The muscles of animals are one of the purest sources. They are high in minerals, and in the case of fish, also high in super healthy fats and oils.

Many other animal based food products yield similar values such as milk and dairy derivatives like cheese, yogurt, and every bodybuilder's favorite—whey protein-based shake.

Plant protein– Even if you're not a vegetarian, a variety of protein sources not only broadens your available resource pool, but it also ensures you get so many other nutrients that you need. Many plants have a surprising amount of protein with the added benefit of fiber, vitamins, and fats that you can't get anywhere else!

Nuts such as almonds and pistachios are great for a high protein snack. They also have lots of healthy fats that support your joints and immunity and help you absorb vitamins and minerals. Most beans combine high fiber with lots of protein. Legumes like peanuts and soybeans are plants that many alternative protein supplements are made from to avoid using animal byproducts. The added bonus of plant protein is that most of them are very low in sugar which helps you to feel full longer.

CARBOHYDRATES

Next up comes the energy abundant carbohydrate. Carbohydrates vary in complexity, but all are made up of strings of glucose molecules. Glucose is sugar. The complexity of the strings of sugars helps determine how long it takes you to digest and prepare those sugars for use as energy. (MedlinePlus 2019)

Sugars– Sugars are the most basic form of carbohydrate. There is some debate on the qualities of sugar—which is best and which is worst—but sugar is sugar, with the exception of modified or manufactured sugars we have created that can have more harmful effects on us. (MedlinePlus 2019)

Sugars provide an immediate and ready form of nourishment for your cells, where little to no work is involved to break them down to use. That's why you get a burst of hyperactivity when you eat an orange or drink a sugary drink, but that energy is often short lived, and not sustainable. Consuming large amounts of sugars can also lead to weight gain, acid reflux, diabetes, and many other long term ailments and damage, so moderation is recommended.

One school of thought among nutritionists on the moderation of sugar consumption is to eat more natural forms of simple sugars, such as fresh fruits and freshly squeezed fruit juices. The drawbacks are that too much simple sugar is not particularly good for you.

Your body's reaction to large amounts of sugar is to release the hormone insulin. This is why you crash so hard after a huge, carb-heavy meal. Insulin released from your pancreas is a direct response to sugar regulation in your body and one of its side effects is drowsiness!

In terms of this *sugar crash*, a more viable solution is to eat more complex carbs which take longer to break down and digest, thus prolonging their energy offering. Many dietitians encourage this while discouraging heavy fruit and snack consumption to lower the intake of overall sugar and dense but fleeting calories in your diet. Another reason for limiting certain fruits is the lack of satiation in fruit sugars. It can make you feel less full and hungry again very quickly, leading to the possibility of overeating.

In contrast to a lot of what we have been taught, sugar is the predominant cause of becoming overweight and obese. While fat can produce fat, particularly in the cases of fried foods and processed oils, our bodies actually store excess energy as fat reserves, so more of the carbs you eat contribute to fat gain than anything else. For this reason, food brand marketing labels can be deceiving by claiming to have low fat while still containing loads of sugar.

Now none of that is to say that you should not ever eat any sugar! Before you go throwing out everything in your pantry, remember that after a hard workout you need to replenish your stores of salts and sugars, as well as your body's water content. Sugary sports drinks do have their place, as do snacks. Many athletes pair a bit of high dextrose candy with their post-workout protein shake for optimal protein absorption.

Starches– Starches are more complex forms of carbs. Starches include root vegetables like potatoes and cereals such as wheat, oats, and rice, and are the primary source of carbohydrates in the human diet. Staple foods of cultures all over the world all center around growing locally specific, starchy, carbohydrate heavy crops due to the high yield of usable food products from most of them.

As far as your modern average diet is concerned, they fall roughly into two categories: processed and unprocessed.

Most *white* starches, or more accurately, *refined starches* have been processed to some degree, such as bleached flour, most rice, and cornstarch. In much the same fashion as simple sugars, refined starches are much easier for our bodies to break down into sugar. The purpose behind these methods mainly has to do with ease of access and usability in cooking and preparation. Unprocessed starches must be heated to absorb water in order to denature the hard surface so they can soften and thicken to eat, whereas processed starches thicken in water instantly. You'll notice the difference in how you can quickly steam white rice, but must boil and simmer whole brown rice for an hour to prepare it. This pre-cooking of starches removes a lot of work on the part of the consumer, but it can simplify the nutritional value of the food and can remove many of the beneficial digestive elements.

As far as unprocessed starches go, cooking is essential to being able to eat them. The process still breaks down the material for digestibility, but fiber and nutrients in the husks cause the starch to digest more slowly, allowing our cells a more sustained and prolonged supply of energy. You will typically feel full for much longer eating these types of starches. When choosing your ingredients, a very basic strategy for recognizing the difference is to check the cooking instructions.

Cereal starches– Cereal grains provide an abundant source of carbohydrates, but these starches tend to also be the most commonly refined. Pasta and breads are super popular examples, and the token phrase you will often find associated with these is *whole grain*, which suggests the cereal was less processed. While there are more healthy options of both, the majority of mass produced products use refined ingredients. Many nutritionists suggest sticking to unprocessed starches when adding these foods to your diet and cooking them yourself. This also limits the amount of preservatives and added salts and sugars.

. . .

Vegetable starches— The most well known vegetable starch is likely the potato. However, there are many options for you if you want to avoid grains and gluten. Peas, corn, yams, spinach, gourds, brussel sprouts, and many other vegetables all provide excellent sources of carbohydrates.

Alternatively, keep in mind that other foods still might contain fair amounts of carbohydrates as well, such as milk and yogurt. This is not inherently a bad thing depending on your goals, but it should be a consideration if you want to limit or increase your carb intake or simply modify the quality of them.

It's pretty safe to say that you should limit your junk food consumption for a variety of reasons, but don't completely eliminate delicious treats from your life! Sometimes a good cheat meal or a cheat day with a big slice of cake can help your mental health.

Fibers— Fiber is another type of complex carbohydrate. Many fibers cannot be broken down to use, which is why you feel fuller longer from high fiber foods and why they can be useful in keeping your digestive track regular and clean by encouraging evacuation. (Gunnars 2018) On the opposite end, pun intended, this is also why too much can cause intestinal distress and cramping, promoting too-frequent excretion.

Because of their digestive properties and carb-curbing nature, fibers can also help lower blood sugar and cholesterol.

Vegetables provide the primary source for most of the fiber in people's diets. Broccoli, avocados, dried fruits, as well as most fruits with edible skins all make the roster for fibrous foods. Potatoes and beans may also be an option when outfitting your diet, depending on your carb allotment.

On the other hand, some surprising snacks can help you stay full and fit like popcorn and nuts. Just be wary of the amount of butter and salt added to these savory treats!

FATS

While fats in food does apply to the organic material, all of us have a layer of fat in varying degrees all over our body and in our muscles. It's also a really good nutrient in food when you get it from the right places!

Fat is an organic compound made of groups of fatty acids. The most common reference to it is animal fat, like ours, which are specifically the type of fat known as triglycerides, or the more vernacular *lipid*.

Fat provides part of the body's source of energy, and is the primary storage of energy—like a battery cell. For this reason, when under stress, you can burn fat in the absence of other energy sources.

Fat is responsible for lubricating joints and insulating our organs from shock. Skin and hair gain their luster from fats, and the layer of tissue insulates us to maintain body temperature.

Our immune system is largely dependent on fat to dilute and isolate bacterial and poisonous intruders in the body, and fat is partially responsible for hormone production in organs and in reducing inflammation. Both of the last two aspects of fat are extremely important for athletes, especially during recovery and growth.

When it comes to eating fat, the nutrient is instrumental in assisting with the digestion and absorption of vitamins and minerals. Home remedies suggest taking a teaspoon of olive oil with your multivitamin for this reason!

Similar to proteins, there are two essential fatty acids we do not synthesize that we need to eat to have. You may have heard them referenced as omega-3 and omega-6 fatty acids. Many brands tote their inclusion as a marketing draw for their product.

You will see certain foods come up again and again as we sculpt our perfect diets due to their diversity and complexity.

These foods are exceptionally good for us, including some *super foods* that provide a huge array of macro and micronutrients. (Wikipedia Contributors 2018)

Avocado is one such food, high in good fats and carbs, with a great amount of protein (for a fruit). Cheese proffers healthy milk fats, unlike some of its fellow milk products which can increase some risks of heart disease when eaten in excess.

Other delicious fat-filled foods include dark chocolate (with low amounts of sugar and dairy added), whole eggs, fatty fish (herring, salmon, sardines, mackerel), nuts, chia seeds, and olive oil. (Gunnars 2017)

WATER

Because our bodies are made up of so much water, as we lose fluids through metabolizing waste and through evaporation, we must replenish our supply or risk dehydration. The exact amount you need is a variable based on your body makeup, climate, temperature, and the activity level you engage in. But, you have to drink some every day or your body will very quickly let you know that it cannot work right without it.

Despite some debate among experts, it is agreed that most people should at least imbibe a liter (around a quart) of water a day. Issues like constipation, cracking skin, and even organ failure can result fairly rapidly from a lack of hydration. (Wikipedia Contributors 2018a)

For all of us sporting individuals, water acts to cool high body temperatures through sweat and drinking. Just be cautious not to let your perception of thirst cause you to overindulge while you are at max output. Our kidneys slow water processing when under duress, so over hydrating is possible in rare cases, resulting in what is basically water poisoning. Definitely a case of too much of a good thing!

MICRONUTRIENTS

Micronutrients are a variety of essential substances we need in very small amounts for proper maintenance and function. While we do receive vast quantities of both in our daily meals, isolating and supplementing our diets with key vitamins and minerals not only promotes better well being, but prevents ailments, diseases, and can boost our performance. ("Vitamins" 2019) Multivitamins usually contain a fairly generalized baseline for common additives, but every person has their own chemical profile that needs to be addressed individually for the best results.

Vitamins– Vitamins are essential chemical compounds mostly found in food that either dissolve in water or fat. Some build up in the body in fat, whereas others pass more quickly through in our water waste, and need to be replenished more frequently. Due to imbalances in our diets, lifestyles, and genetics, most humans have insufficiencies of some vitamin or another. As such, the advancement of vitamin research has developed into the biggest supplemental market for our diets to fill those gaps in nutrition. Leave yourself a note to remember to take your vitamins!

Minerals– Minerals are inorganic elements that compose our physical makeup. Much like vitamins, these elements are necessary in minuscule quantities for preserving our health and sustaining biological processes. Calcium helps maintain bone density, for example, while potassium keeps your kidneys working. The electrolyte sodium is perhaps the most well known mineral that we ingest every day. It's salt!

. . .

Antioxidants– Antioxidants are any vitamin, nutrient, or protein that help expel toxins from waste byproducts and foreign reactive oxygen species that accumulate in the body over time. Vitamins A, C, and E are all antioxidants. (Newman 2020)

Each of these terms we've reviewed are a science and field of study in and of themselves, so don't expect to become an expert overnight. This information is the first stepping stone toward mastery. We are here to get you on track identifying your needs and optimizing your performance. But, before we move forward, we have to take a quick look back at how we got to where we are in sports nutrition today.

CHAPTER 3
NUTRITION HISTORY

Never underestimate the benefits of a good stretch! Lengthening the muscle is the only way to push through plateaus and keep your joints and tendons as flexible as you need them to be. While you're at it, stretch out your mind as we toe-touch on a few of the discoveries and achievements in human sciences that built the spectacular body of sports nutrition knowledge we have to assist us today. Without the astounding flexibility of the human brain we would never have come this far!

A BIT OF HISTORY

Sports nutrition, also called exercise nutrition, is the modern study and practice of diet optimization to improve and maintain performance in sports and exercise, whether professional or otherwise. ("Sports Nutrition, Definition, Purpose, History, Description" n.d.)

It also incorporates the correlation with *exercise physiology* to better understand how the body moves, works, and what it needs to function based on its action. This distinction of terminology comes with the more recent inclusion of many less physical competitions in the world of sporting events such as poker and chess. That doesn't mean that sports nutrition cannot also help those competitors eat right for their mental acuity!

It may come as a shock to learn that so much of what we know now has only just been comprehensively studied within the last forty years or so. Prior to the 1980s, sports science, medicine, and nutrition were fairly rudimentary, and all together disparate without the specialization we have today. Rather, the study of athletes centered more around *exercise physiology*.

To us, a lot of the conclusions and established fields seem pretty straight forward now, but nutrition and physiology, much like the overall medical sciences they're rooted in, have gone through massive paradigm shifts over the last hundred and fifty years. We would consider much of what was practiced even a hundred years ago pseudoscience at best. Unfortunately, the scientific and medical fields have had a history of closely guarded access and deeply ingrained tradition, and even an unsettling amount of superstition. You may find it unsettling and even horrifying that physical health and natural science were not always considered the same study!

From drinking alcohol and other stimulants for energy, to snake-oil salesman type remedies, fear, tradition, and pride all factored into the misinformation and widely accepted notions in the early days of sport sciences. Much of the experimentation dealt in trial and error and how things 'felt' as opposed to what was actually happening inside the body. This slow and tedious development is also because, as we now know, sport science is and has to be chained to the development of its parents in anatomy, nutrition, mental health (which is still a burgeoning field with many hurdles yet to overcome), and general medicinal treatment. They are one and the same.

Adjacently, part of the issue with sluggish advancement had to do with available means and perception of importance. Between wars and global disease outbreaks, industrial advancement paved the way for comfort entertainment and free time to begin to become part of the working peoples' lives, and as education became more readily available to more people, more focus could be placed on developing new fields of study and new venues of competitive sporting events. Teams and aspiring competitors largely drawn from after-work amateurs would evolve into full time careers, and with money involved, inevitable progress could be made.

EARLY NUTRITION

While we have a few examples in ancient records of athletes recording their diets or mentioning their regimens, it wasn't until the mid 1800s that any real scholarly medical study began on the physiology of exercise. Even then, real research and substantial strides were not actually made until the turn of the century as the subject gained a little traction with established schools of study surrounding nutrition and exercise.

Right around 1900 is the first time we see things like nutrient values of proteins established and promoted through emerging governmental organizations. This informative programming through government agencies sought to start health education among the general populace alongside growing scholastic opportunities and eventual mandatory education for all children. (Mozaffarian, Rosenberg, and Uauy 2018)

As it often happens, war fuels discovery and often controls the provision of those discoveries.

In the US for example, most information published to distribute information about food health and safety came from the military and tied in very closely with the looming current event of World War I. The prominent motive behind the material provided to citizens dealt with disease prevention from tainted food stock and health maintenance through a good diet.

Subsequently, in most of the early dietary education of the common man, the major focus of nutritional information provided by many governments dealt more with the safe storage and safe handling of food, and only touched on the bare necessities of balancing a diet with varied food groups. This also veered heavily toward limiting food waste, maximizing food storage longevity, and accumulating stock to mitigate shortages during war time and economic depressions.

BUILDING BENCHMARKS

Alongside the discoveries being made in other scientific fields, nutritional science truly began to develop in the early 1900s. It was now seen outside of the simple reasons we eat to sate hunger, to more of the function of the elements involved in the foods and how they affected our bodies. This included the discovery of micronutrients in the form of vitamins.

So as we see the first vitamin isolated and studied, we can hop ahead a few decades and witness it synthesized for the first time, opening up an entire field of research to cure deficiency related diseases. A few more decades into the 60s and we have isolated every vitamin and mineral leading to the birth of the multivitamin industry today. (Mozaffarian, Rosenberg, and Uauy 2018)

Jump back over to Europe in the 1930s, and we see some of the first carbohydrate and fat metabolism studies in Sweden. This was an early look at another focus that could develop once vitamin and mineral deficiencies had been largely addressed through the fortification of foods and supplementation of commonly purchased goods: sugar and dietary fats. (Andati, Bryan 2018)

Somewhere in the midst of that, again, another world war set the narrative for food study and rationing. Despite the possibly biased promotion of convenient, cheap, abundant provisions to help navigate feeding armies and citizens, one very long-lasting dietary fact emerged out of the 40s. Calories in should equal calories out.

So we leap back to the 1960s once more and you progress into studies on muscular energy storage in Scandinavia. 1965 rolls around and we get what is probably the most known sports food product today—Gatorade! ("Origins and History of Sport Nutrition" n.d.)

In the 1970s, universities began to develop programs for exercise studies, particularly in the US. Most of this early physical research began with runners, as running could be replicated in a stationary form to monitor, and long endurance athletes tended to suffer more from depleted stores of energy. The military, including growing space programs across the globe, needed to employ the latest methods and find new techniques to train their people to be in the best condition to survive the hardest conditions possible. (Daniels and Hanson 2021)

Throughout all of this, muscle building was growing into a sport of its own, despite negative views in *real* sports toward the "circus sideshow" strong man stereotype. Nutritionally, protein that helps create all of those muscles was also sidelined due to the difficult nature of isolating where to start. Proteins exist all throughout our bodies and protein synthesis is much more difficult to simulate than sugars and fats.

Strides in muscular and strength development were left to those sidelined muscle men to experiment through trial and error. The trend would continue for several decades as competition and ambition demanded ever-loftier goals.

From the 70s into the 80s, cooperation between institutions helped to begin deciphering exactly how much of certain things we need, but this butted up against the hurdle of determining which foods would provide the best means of that delivery. And so, sports nutrition was officially born in the mid-80s. Nutritionists, and their application in sports, emerged as a new specialized field to help translate the science of food and exercise physiology into practical application.

Simple views about categorizing athletes began to change shortly after. Previously, athletes either fell into endurance athletes or strength athletes. This all paired neatly with the nutritional habit of the endurance athletes eating primarily carbs for endurance, and strength athletes primarily protein for strength. They weren't totally wrong, just limited in the scope of their vision and missing some pieces to the puzzle.

It is pretty hard to believe that it wasn't until the 90s that athletes began to incorporate exercises from outside their sport into their training. Resistance training worked its way into just about every sport-training camp, and aerobic regimens filled out power-based sport programs. Coupled with ever-refining nutrition implementation, suddenly athletes were beginning to be able to train longer and harder than ever before, fueled by the right kinds of foods and supplements and varying the workloads into a balance across their physique.

We really get the best of it now. With all of this exponentially evolving knowledge available to us, we can raise the bar of our achievements even further and push our bodies to greater echelons of perfection.

And speaking of bodies, it's time to take a closer look at the incredible machine that makes all of this possible. We've all got one—the human body!

PART TWO
BODY OF WORK

CHAPTER 4
PHYSIQUE

Physique, in its most basic definition, is the natural physical structure of a human body. ("Definition of PHYSIQUE." 2022) Think of the famous DaVinci design of the Vitruvian man diagram as a reference. The image outlines an ideal of bodily proportions and a general interpretation of a human's layout. This is a very relative concept, from a very long time ago, but it represents a good place to start in understanding how to see your body and its outer functionality.

Along this line of thinking, we use other, similar ways to look at our physique. Terms used frequently to describe body types and shapes include *figure*, which gives us more of a fashionable vibe, or *frame*, that connotes a bit more of how we carry ourselves while in motion. *Constitution* denotes a sense of what we are made up of, perhaps in our muscular appearance and where we tend to carry our body fat. Very much in the same tone, you might hear a trainer reference your *build*. All of these are useful for relating and understanding where you are and where you want to be, but they don't effectively convey your athleticism.

In bodybuilding competitions, the term is a system or method of rating competitors and their musculature. This is getting closer to serving our needs. For nutritional and athletic purposes, we need to look at rating our physique more in the terms of physical fitness and what level you are at relative to your diet and muscular development. An *athletic physique* is largely considered a muscular, lean, low-fat-percentage body. Be that as it may, within every sport, the term applies differently based on the demands of that sport. That means that not everyone will, or should, strive for this look. Primarily, you should aspire to a healthy physique first, then see to the gains you need to make to compete at the optimal level.

Some people are born with a propensity for a more athletic build. Others must attain it through difficult training. Nevertheless, all sports performers must work to maximize their body in aspects that compliment their activity.

BODY TYPES

In the 1940s, Dr. William Sheldon submitted the idea of body types that he called *somatotypes*. This categorization method was designed to accommodate the various shapes humans come in and their tendencies. These body types have dominant traits, benefits, and weaknesses, but they do not necessarily delegate a person's capacity for fitness. Trainers and nutritionists have used these categorizations to establish general benchmarks and recognize how to help people enhance their physique. Just to be clear, anyone with any body type can develop athleticism.

Almost every person can be placed in one of the three main categories: endomorphs, ectomorphs, and mesomorphs. Most of us roughly fall into one of these brackets, but like we said, it is a generalization. ("Athletic Body Type: Getting into the Nitty Gritty of Attaining This Body Shape" 2021)

Endomorphs– Endomorphs naturally have more curves, a thicker build, and a higher body fat content. This body type finds it easy to gain both muscle and fat, and difficult to lose weight. People of this build need to watch their caloric intake and most importantly, watch their sugar and fat levels, as they tend to accumulate fat easily. With higher fat levels, making sure to monitor insulin sensitivity through lower sugar intake will make gaining or losing weight a much healthier task.

Ectomorphs– This type is leaner—skinny even—with low muscle mass and very little fat on the body. Ectomorphs commonly have longer limbs. They struggle with gaining any substantial weight, muscle, or fat. This body type is often considered to have a high metabolism. Getting sufficient and balanced nutrients will be essential for the ectomorph as they can eat more without much effect. Loading up on healthy foods will prevent an overload of bad cholesterol and artery clogging bad fats. Just because they're skinny, doesn't mean they are immune to these things.

Ecto-endomorph– This is a combinational category used to describe the pear-shaped figure. Ecto-endos will have a thin upper body and a thicker lower half. Their advantages and struggles with fat/muscle gains follow suit. Most weight gain will occur in the lower extremities. Mobility can become an issue in extreme cases, so this body type should be mindful of weight gain and its effects on their lower body.

Endo-ectomorphs– Endo-ectos have the opposite combination of top and bottom predispositions. They carry more weight on the upper half of the body and struggle to gain weight on their legs. People with this inclination need to be careful about upper body fat levels for heart health and other major organ functions.

. . .

Mesomorphs– Some consider this the most naturally athletic build because of balance. They are a more neutral and average body type. Characteristics of a mesomorph include a medium build, higher muscle profile, and an even distribution of fat. Weight gain occurs evenly in fat or muscle across the entire body. The even distribution of fat and muscle does not exempt mesomorphs from unhealthy consequences of poor diet or a lack of exercise.

Now, these are mostly aesthetic terms, more visually based to identify characteristics, but they can help you find where to start. Just basing your assessments of yourself on these types cannot tell you how athletic you actually are, but recognizing your strengths and weaknesses is integral to planning a training regimen and diet. Common traits in those somatotypes will give you useful guidance in knowing what foods typically work better for someone of your constitution.

Using every tool at your disposal, you can increase your athleticism and change your body while catering to your body type's needs. Strength and endurance testing will give you a better gauge of athleticism, and you should never underestimate the benefits of consulting a professional trainer to assess your current state.

On that note, let's take a look at the human body!

ANATOMY

Your body is the entire focus for all of your nutritional study, as well as the source of all of your athletic output. Understanding the inner workings is essential to understanding the resulting action and what the demands you put on your body do to it. It's also instrumental in telling you why you aren't able to accomplish something or why your body is not responding well to what you're asking of it. There may be a deficit in your diet that needs addressing!

Skeleton– I think everyone is pretty familiar with the human skeleton. It's your support beam structure. You know—your bones!

Muscles– Muscles are systems of contractile tissue that we use to move. There are three types: smooth muscle (non-striated), cardiac muscle, and skeletal muscle (striated). Striated muscles are attached directly to your skeleton, and make up the majority of the muscles in the body. We use these powerful fibers like levers and pulleys against the structure of our bone frame to move and exert force. (Milner 2008)

Cardiac muscle is a specialized, striated muscle fiber, but unlike skeletal muscle it is not a voluntary system. Your autonomous system keeps your heart beating without any conscious thought. (Milner 2008) That's a good thing. (You can, however, learn to regulate your pulse through training, but that is more about disciplining your mind and reactions than anything else.)

Non-striated muscle is all of the other muscular tissue that lines organs and connects internal tissues. It is also run by the auto-nervous system. ("Muscle | Systems, Types, Tissue, & Facts" 2019)

Key nutrients to ensure muscle maintenance and growth:

- Water—it carries nutrients to your muscles.

- Lean protein—amino acids create more muscle and heal muscle.
- Magnesium, calcium, and potassium. All of these minerals prevent cramping and aid in muscle relaxation and assist other nutrient consumption.
- Vitamin D promotes testosterone, the key hormone for muscular development.
- Carbs will replenish glycogen stores in the muscle and give you energy for work.
- Iron and vitamin B-12 carry oxygen to your muscles. (Ayuda 2018)

Muscle groups in human anatomical description are classified by location on the body and appearance. For example, the quadriceps femoris, the four-muscle-group on the front of your thigh, is attached to the femur bone of your upper leg.

Musculature– Musculature describes the layout of the muscles of your body or can be used to refer to a specific part of the body. All animals, including us, have musculature. This is only important to note the difference between muscle and musculature as we begin to discuss your performance and development. ("Definition of MUSCULATURE" 2022)

Fat– Fat, or *adipose tissue*, is connective tissue that serves a whole bunch of purposes that we have already mentioned in the previous chapters, at least in passing. Fat is technically considered an organ because of its involvement in energy storage and its functional role in hormone production. The tissue can become harmful to us in excessive amounts built up from disorders, inactivity, or excessive food consumption. (Wikipedia Contributors 2019g)

Fat percentage in the body over a certain amount, which differs for everyone, can lead to inflammation and many health concerns. Too much fat can wear down the body and put undue strain on the joints and tendons, and can put stress on the muscular systems. Chemically, it can cause a host of problems and illnesses, interrupting organ function.

It does serve a very important purpose for our health by insulating our temperature, as well as padding organs from shock and serving to store long term reserves of cell energy.

Macronutrient ratios have been shown to have little effect on the depletion of fat in weight loss programs. More important is the quantity of calories eaten and the quality of those calories. Limiting sugars and choosing healthy fats and leaner proteins hold a much higher value in improved health. ("Fat Facts" 2021)

Nutrients that promote healthy fat levels:

- Sufficient protein will promote fat burn, more satiety, and help you feel full longer.
- Whole grains break down slower for sustained energy and insulin balance.
- Good fats, monounsaturated and polyunsaturated fat (found in nuts, avocados, seeds and oils) improve cholesterol and decrease inflammation.

Joints– Joints are where bones meet and connect. Joints and cartilaginous tissue are the hinges responsible for all of our abilities to move. Flexibility and longevity of your specialized synovial joints will play a huge factor in your sport mastery. These are the movement joints like knees and elbows. Do not count out the other bones and their connections. Our structure is a sum of all of its parts. (Colby College. 2013)

For bone and joint support make sure you are getting enough:

- Calcium for blood circulation and bone density.
- Omega-3 fatty acids for reduced swelling responses.
- Vitamin D for calcium absorption.
- Antioxidants from dark red and purple fruits block certain reactive proteins, limiting inflammation in joints. ("Eight Essential Nutrients" 2022)

Ligaments and Tendons– These two words get thrown around a lot in tandem. They do have a lot to do with each other, but they are different tissues.

Ligaments connect the bones across the joint and prevent contrary movement against the natural motion of the hinge. Without getting too technical, there are various types of tissues within the joint that function differently in individual joints like cartilage and bursae. The short version is that these all serve to protect the joint and keep it moving right. They also provide padding for impact and damage prevention. This tissue can be worn down over time, and, in some cases, it is not replenished by the body.

Tendons, on the other hand (and in both of your hands!), are the elastic bands that help the muscle push and pull against the bone to activate a desired movement or force. Strengthening your tendons is just as (or more) important as strengthening your muscles. Muscles adapt quickly, tendons do not. As such, slow progression and repetition are key in resistance training to allow the tendons time to build and strengthen. Stretching and keeping them flexible is equally important. If you lengthen and build your muscles without stretching and strengthening your tendons to match, you will inevitably set yourself up for injury.

To keep your tendons and ligaments in great health get plenty of:

- Protein keeps coming up, but it is essential for all repairs!
- Vitamins A and E for cell repair. Vitamin E prevents symptoms of tendinitis.
- A solid mineral profile in your dietary vitamin supplement.

("Nutrition for Tendon and Ligament Health" 2016)

BMI (BODY MASS INDEX)

BMI is a system of measurement taken from the mass and height of a person. Mass being the muscle, bone, and fat compared to the stature of a person. The basic figure was designed using kilograms and meters: your weight divided by your height squared:

- BMI= kb/m^2
- BMI= $(lbs \times 703)/(height\ in\ inches^2)$

This system was proposed for assessing percentages of fat to muscle ratios and baseline health statistics for the general populace. As with many of the other tools available to the average amateur athlete, its universal application offers a broad window to understanding your composition. It is a useful tool for goal setting, and estimated progress tracking. Several medical and health websites offer a BMI calculator and charts for you to get an idea of where you stand. (CDC 2019)

Statistically, this system provides medical specialists with a decent gauge of your health, whether the number is too high or low. Both eventualities are associated with higher occurrences of health issues and risks of certain illnesses and mortality.

Consulting a specialist and having tests done will give a more detailed profile of your ratios.

Other methods of measuring your body fat include a Body Fat Caliper, or an Electrical Impedance Myography device installed in many consumer weight products—either of which can be acquired easily online. These devices typically have a margin of error between three and five percent body fat.

The only way to increase the accuracy in measuring your body fat content is to have a professional test done using X-rays or hydrostatic measurement comparison, and in the most effective case, a combination of multiple techniques. This is what is called the multi-compartment model. It comes down to whether you really need to know your fat percentage or not. If an estimate will work, go the cheap and easy route.

YOU ARE WHAT YOU EAT

Nutrition plays a vital role in developing the physique you want. Dietitians and trainers will often use the expression that weight loss and physical fitness is "80% diet and 20% exercise." Some argue that it's 100% of both! ("Why Sticking to 80% Diet" 2018)

These numbers aren't exactly quantifiable in reality, but it's the concept behind the statement that matters. Of the two, nutrition has the most immediate effectual ramifications on your body.

The math is simple. You eat far more often than you exercise. Even if you were to train twice a day, seven days a week, you would still eat more times than you would train. And to be fair, in that specific, pro-athlete-like example, you would indelibly be burning incredible quantities of calories and would need to be eating constantly! For example, Michael Phelps spent about six hours per day in training and ate between 6-10,000 calories a day preparing for the Olympics! ("Michael Phelps' 10000" 2021)

The fact is, you cannot eat poorly and excessively and make the progress you want. No amount of exercise will out-burn too many calories or foods that cause damage to the body. (Leal 2015)

So, in case the balance of the two parts of the subject wasn't clear enough, look at it this way: you can lose weight and improve health ONLY by dieting and not changing your activity level. Of course, exercise is extremely important to a healthy lifestyle both mentally and physically, but it goes to show how imperative your diet and nutrition are. Fortunately, you are an athlete, so you're already on the right track.

So far, this has been a lot of information to absorb. Nevertheless, each bit of knowledge will help you formulate your plan to be the best, at every milestone on your journey, whether it be at the amateur or expert level.

CHAPTER 5
MUSCLE FUNCTION

In this chapter we finally get started into the sports-half of the equation and how the various abilities of our amazing bodies activate to allow for competition and exercise. When push comes to shove, it takes more than just pushing and pulling to transform your body. You have to change the way you think. Your mental game, in addition to your physique, will play a huge role in your dieting and discipline.

But don't get me wrong, the pulling and pushing are very important!

PUSHING AND PULLING

Our muscles have specific directives and paths they move along. You'll remember the comparison we made earlier about how your muscles and tendons work like a system of pulleys and levers, pushing and pulling against your skeleton to create force. Each muscle and group have movement patterns we follow to work out both individual muscles, and in most cases, teaming up multiple muscles into compound movements. ("Push-Pull Workouts" 2020)

. . .

Push muscles– The chest, or pectoral muscles and the quadriceps that make up the front of your thigh are the two dominant muscle groups in *pushing* force generation. Squats and push ups or bench press are essential examples of how those two groups work. Most of the exercises associated with pushing focus heavily on exerting force away from the body with a few exceptions like the pec flye which incorporates the alternate range of motion of the chest inwards, but even this is sometimes misinterpreted, as the pushing force is simply redirected across the body, not actually toward it.

Complimenting those powerful muscles are the minor pushing muscles which all act in concert or support the major muscles. The triceps, calves, and, in an indirect way, the lower back and sacrum lend their outward drive to almost every major pushing move we do. They can be isolated in training, and should be, but there are few movements we can make that don't activate some other muscle—even just for stability.

Pulling muscles– The back consists of 20 muscle pairs along the spine and almost every one of them functions to give us our upper body pulling force. For the sake of simplicity and reference, we can mostly just say *lats* to sum up the biggest visible form in the posterior silhouette. Just the act of standing requires a constant pull against the fulcrum of our hips and waist to keep us upright! Obviously, this system of muscles being so intricately laced into our neck, shoulders, ribs, spine and pelvis is a highly complicated machine that we will not dissect in graphic detail here, but you get the idea.

Moving down the body, the gluteal muscles, more commonly called the buttocks muscles, make up the strongest muscle group in the body. These muscles are also the longest length of any in your body. Standing upright and locomotion would not be possible without the use of the gluteal muscles. Their function also serves in direct response to most of your quad pushing motion, recoiling to help you drive the force of your legs out. That's why your rear end feels as sore as your thighs after leg presses or squats.

In action, we will henceforth focus on what most training plans outline in terms of grouping. Pushing muscles and exercises will fall into:

- Pecs (chest)
- Front delts (shoulders)
- Triceps (back of the arms)
- Quads (front of the thighs)
- Calves (generally an auxiliary muscle and isn't always isolated as it functions in all leg workouts)

Pulling muscles and their exercises will group as:

- Lats (back)
- Hamstrings (back of the thighs)
- Glutes
- Biceps (front of the arms)
- Forearms and shins can be isolated as well for strengthening (considered auxiliary as well)

("The Push/Pull/Legs Routine for Muscle Gains | Aston University" 2016)

IN PRACTICE

Related to talk of pushing and pulling in the previous chapter, you may have heard of a *push/pull workout plan* in passing. This type of training is a good example to demonstrate what we are looking at and how most muscle groups have an antagonistic counterpart. Push/pull training contrasts opposing movements of muscles and pairs them in sets to optimize workload for time. For example, in the normal break you would give your triceps to recover from the set of push-downs you just did, you can work in a set of bicep curls. Because of the somewhat independent nature of these two muscles sitting back to back against your humerus bone and glycogen storage in your muscles, while one muscle is fatigued and burning from pushing, the other can be pulling, saving you time and ultimately increasing the overall workload on your body in a shorter span. This can also activate an aerobic response through intensity, adding a cardiovascular aspect to your resistance training.

COMPOUND MOVEMENTS

As we mentioned above, muscles working in concert are what trainers call *compound exercises*. Not only do these movements incorporate various groups to achieve force, but they serve broader benefits to actual functions in everyday life, as well as in sporting endeavors. It is highly unlikely that you would ever just use one muscle in any sport, so the integration of more muscles into play builds coordination and all of the connective tissue and tendons that bind each system to the others. ("What Are Compound Exercises?" 2021)

Compound exercises are the best moves for beginners to build foundational strength and ability. Coordination at the start will lead to big gains later and avoid injuries down the line.

In some routines, compound exercises can save you time and tend to burn more calories. Additionally, they offer dynamic stretching in your movements and increase active flexibility.

Some examples of compound exercises:

- Squats incorporate glutes, quads, hamstrings, calves, hip flexors, and the back to stabilize.
- Deadlifts incorporate your entire posterior chain from your neck down to your heels!
- Pushups incorporate your full arm and shoulder to help the pectoral push.
- Pullups share arm use with the entire back and a tense core. Even though you are dragging your legs as dead weight, you still need to keep them in check so they don't hinder your pull.
- Planks require tension in the arms, legs, and core, including your abdominals and the lower back muscles. This one is a full posture exercise.

("What Are Compound Exercise | AFA Blog" 2018)

Additionally, compound exercises can mean combining two moves into one exercise like in the case of the power clean. The move starts with an explosive deadlift, but turns into a brief upright row, ultimately ending in an overhead press. This is a prime example of maximum effort for time in one exercise.

ISOLATION MOVEMENTS

While compound movement tends to grow your overall solidity and a balanced command of your body, isolating individual muscles and joint movements becomes more and more important as you increase your athleticism and require more specialized tasks from your body. Focusing on a single muscle or muscle group is used for targeting elements of your musculature you want to improve both visually and functionally without stressing other muscles in the process. It can also be used to help recover from injury as developmental therapy by working around the damaged

areas to still maintain healthy activity. ("How to Use Common Isolation Exercises" 2021)
Great examples of isolation exercises:

- Pec flys and crossovers are an effective tool for singling out your chest, which is one of the more difficult muscles to isolate due to its linkage to so many other muscle systems.
- Forward or side lateral raises activate all three muscles in your deltoid, or shoulder muscle.
- Any variation of bicep curls develop the paired muscles on the front of your arm.
- Quad extensions target the two parts of the muscles right above the knee, but also activate up into the center to help give you that tear drop definition.
- Hamstring curls act just like a bicep curl, highlighting your hamstring's concentric ability.

("Compound vs. Isolation Exercises" 2018)
Push/pull routines often rely on isolation pairings that consolidate your time. Think about trying to alternate sets between some opposing muscle groups when doing isolation workouts. (i.e. Barbell bicep curls alternated with triceps kickbacks)

HYPERTROPHY

Hypertrophy occurs in any muscle when you exhaust it through repetitions, but isolation exercises can be a go-to form of achieving that glorious burning sensation you get from pushing your body hard in specific areas. That threshold of burnout in your muscles is caused by lactic acid building up as you force the muscle to use energy to create force, leading to fermentation in the muscle. It sounds a little uncomfortable, but this is natural! You need those chemical reactions to grow. Just make sure you drink plenty of water to stay hydrated, as this will help flush out the acids produced in your workout and allow the muscle to bounce back more quickly. (And eat lots of protein to fuel muscle growth!)

Be mindful of overusing isolation movements, as they can cause imbalances. In other words, don't spend too much time developing one muscle group while the rest of your body falls behind! Some exercises are more fun and more satisfying than others, but if it's hard, that means you are weak in that area and should be working on it! Furthermore, imbalances can lead to a false sense of strength that can lead to injury of the neglected parts of your body.

ENDURANCE

As you increase your strength through isolating areas, you can also increase the length of time you can use those muscles. ("Endurance" 2020) This is endurance, sometimes called stamina.

There are some nuances between stamina and endurance if we want to get technical. Endurance is basically your body's longevity of exertion at a certain activity. Stamina is often used to include the idea of how you feel during the activity, your mental energy as well as your muscular fatigue. More accurately, stamina is the idea of how long your muscles can work at near maximum effort. (Yetman 2020)

Think of it this way: stamina will tell you how many times you could perform a task in a specific amount of time, while endurance will tell you how long you could maintain a given pace.

Regardless of the subtle definitions, they are part of the same idea. It's all about energy storage, how efficiently you use that energy in your muscles, and the strength of your joints and tendons in their fortitude and tolerance of extended workloads.

Your mind has a lot to do with endurance. Mental stress can

cause you to fail just as easily as getting tired. Learning to subdue your instinctive aversion to discomfort will play a huge role in growing your endurance. Eventually, you won't even notice the pain!

Just remember to always be very honest with yourself about that pain. There is a distinct difference between growing pain and injury. Listen to your body!

There are a huge variety of methods to increase your endurance depending on your goals and what type of activity you want to accomplish. Endurance training can lead to some loss of endurance strength and power, so consider keeping a resistance training element in your routine to round out your workouts.

The SAID principle (Specific Adaptation to Imposed Demands) can be applied to every type of workout, but endurance training reflects the meaning pointedly: Whatever you do, your body responds to and makes adjustments accordingly.

Overloading is another good way to raise your threshold. As you adapt, you must raise volume, duration, or your level of effort (e.g. increasing your running speed).

STRENGTH

The first thing that comes to mind for a lot of people when we think of strength are the chiseled and massive figures of Ronnie Coleman or Arnold Schwarzenegger. Strongman competitions display incredible feats of power and muscular prowess. Football linebackers plow into each other and slam unlucky opponents to the turf—all excellent examples of human strength in action!

Physical strength is our ability to execute a task by generating force. ("Physical Strength" 2020) A slightly more scientific view of strength is our exertion of force over objects. Strength training raises that level of potential exertion. It amounts to how many muscle fibers you can recruit to a task and how intensely you recruit them. Through training you will create more muscle fiber density which results in more available recruitment and output. It's a lot like adding resistance bands to your exercises. The more bands you link together in your muscles, the more tension you can create which translates into more energy to move things. ("Physical Strength: Why" 2020)

Strength branches out into every physical activity in different ways:

- Raw power or force, called *absolute strength*, applies to lifting heavy weights, pulling a car. Maximum output!
- Explosive strength deals in fast twitch muscle fibers that respond more quickly. Bursting into a sprint requires this type of strength. Lifting a weight off the ground and the initial pull is explosive strength.
- Relative strength is proportional to your body like gymnastics and performing any exercise involving moving yourself through space.
- Strength endurance ties its capacity for repetition in resistance.

("Understanding the 4 Types of Strength" 2020)

Generally, a slow and steady method is the only long term successful approach to gaining any strength and building long lasting muscle fiber. While your training may be intense, your body can only grow so fast. Progressively upping the intensity and changing the types of exercises you do is a very effective way to challenge your muscles and gain strength.

As we get into details later in the book, we will discuss different methods of training you can try to achieve your desired outcome.

FLEXIBILITY

Stiffness is likely the sensation most of us are more familiar with than flexibility. The two are complementary concepts. The less stiff you can become, the more flexible you will be. Likewise, if you work on your flexibility, you will be stiff far less often. ("Stiffness" 2022)

Flexibility affects sports and activities by developing your reach, response, and your capacity to supersede your limits. And, of course, there are sports that are only possible due to increased flexibility, such as gymnastics and ice skating. ("Flexibility | Sports Medicine" 2014)

The compliance of a surface or object defines how much it can give before it breaks or is damaged. And that's not really an analogy, that's how your muscles and tendons work. Flexibility resides within the pain free range of motion of a joint or muscle system. ("Stiffness" 2022)

Several factors can compromise the integrity of joint motion:

- Injury from accidents or unsafe exercise form
- Disuse
- Misuse and overuse can cause damage and a wearing down
- Fatigue leads to compromising form

Stretching– Stretching after workouts is important for recovery but also for growth and decreased risk of injury. It equates to maintenance for both muscle and tendons. Other benefits of flexibility training and upkeep include coordination, proper muscle recoil and response, and better blood flow.

Make sure that when you stretch, use even distribution,

stretching all over, not just problem spots or strong spots. Warming up before stretching prepares the area with blood, priming the muscles and joints to awaken. Blood flow will help avoid strains or pulls.

Static stretching– This stretch is held for a length of time. It takes the brain about 30 seconds to fully recognize and understand a stretch, so give it at least that long to settle in. Therapists recommend one to two minutes a day of stretching for all areas.

Dynamic stretching– *Dynamic* implies stretching in motion. It could mean a combination of warm up/stretching like leg swings or jumping jax that take the muscles and joints through a range of motion. Many trainers employ it during workouts and movement as well, encouraging you to go deeper into the motion to get the little stretch at the bottom or top of a move.

Subtle and smooth movements can be added during a stretch to explore the range of a joint and broaden the scope of the stretch and its effectiveness. Apply such moves gently.

BALANCE

It may come as a surprise that balance more than any other physical fitness attribute is imperative for our coordination and ability. Frankly, without it we would not be able to do the rest.

Balance is the biomechanical function of operating in gravity. It is inherent in us, but also a skill that can be developed. You likely do not remember learning to stand as a baby or to walk, but you had the tools and capacity and developed the ability. ("Balance" 2022)

Natural movements in the body from breathing and staying on our feet cause sway and tilt, and we react to them instinctively. Our sensorimotor control and perception has a lot to do with it. To maintain and regulate balance, we use our eyes for linear points of reference. We also use sensations in our spinal movement and our feet of what is around us and what surfaces we are on or can touch. Equilibrium is our built in perception of forces applied to us. ("How to Maintain and Improve Physical Balance" 2018)

To use a simple analogy, just look at a construction level. The bubble always tells you if something is straight. Our inner ear and vestibular system work to determine our level. Upsetting the liquid in that system causes disorientation. This is why we get dizzy from rapid motion.

Part of balance training is becoming accustomed to those sensations and understanding when our senses are confused. Then, reacting how we know we should, not how we feel we should, thereby suppressing our auto response.

Training can include:

- Strengthening the core with balance-challenging yoga
- Coordination exercises
- Line drills

Your central nervous system can become impaired when fatigued and lead to an inability to balance. When you are exhausted you'll note that you can feel wobbly or off balance. Likewise, in competitive sports, balance is a key factor in determining the effects of concussions or fitness to perform. Often, athletes insist on continuing despite these signs, either from ambition or in many cases effects of imbalance impairing their perception of their own state. Treatment plans for recovery of many injuries often start or heavily integrate balance to regain normal function. ("The Importance of Good Physical Balance" 2016)

This chapter is only an overview of everything involved in body movement, but it gives you a good basis to move forward on. There are entire books dedicated to each of the subjects we have discussed so far. Hopefully, this information will spark your interest in expanding your knowledge about your body.

Next, we need to address one last important part of that body—the brain.

CHAPTER 6
MENTAL HEALTH AND COMPETITIVE SPORTS

Possibly the most important aspect of exercise and our daily lives is mental health. We won't start spouting inspirational quotes here, mind you. This isn't that kind of self help book!

An athletic frame of mind will be addressed in depth in the sequel to this book. We aim to make you a master of your diet first, before we move on to higher thinking! Since your mind is in charge of learning and implementing all of the nutritional expertise you gain, we do need a chapter on it to at least give you the rundown.

The idea of achieving a higher state of mind in Zen meditation is great, no question, but short of mastering those techniques, your mind still controls everything you do. Every reaction you make, when to do something and when not to, is the exclusive responsibility of your brain. You have to make the best decisions with the information and stimuli you have. That sounds an awful lot like sports, doesn't it? Life is constantly placing hurdles and obstacles in your path that you have to mitigate, dodge, or overcome. The metaphorical comparisons of your life and sports sounds a bit cheesy, but it is a good analogy.

In the chapters dealing with sport related training we will discuss some parts of the mental game needed to achieve higher levels of performance. These can include meditation and other mental disciplines.

MIND YOUR MIND

Your brain is a muscle that needs to be worked out. Exercising your mind is a realm unto itself, but you will train your brain as you train your body and vice versa. The two are inseparably interwoven. Stress management comes from healthy exercise, but is ultimately handled by the brain. You have to make decisive and meaningful steps to address and sustain your state of well being.

Mental drive and discipline must be cultivated with your natural competitiveness to give you the motivation you need to succeed. You are the only one who can make anything happen for yourself. Staying present in the moment and being conscious of how you are now will help you immensely.

Stay aware of these aspects of your thought process using your presence of mind:

- Self assessing your state of well being. Aches, pains, tension. What is causing it? Have I had enough water today? What have I eaten?
- Mind-body connection, being aware of what is going on inside you as well as around you. Monitor spikes in emotion as well as energy swells and flags.
- Refuse to be negligent. It's all too easy to ignore behaviors and influences that are detrimental to your health! Take care of yourself. Maintaining regular self care is easier than starting and stopping.

Eating to feed your working mind is essential to brain function and performance. There are also foods that can help you stay alert and focused as you train your brain.

- Try low sugar, high fiber foods for long stints of concentration. Your body will burn a lot of calories when you are thinking intensely. Granola and other slow digesting carbs can help.
- Coffee not only provides caffeine for alertness and concentration, but antioxidants that may be linked to lowering risks of neurological diseases.
- Blueberries contain anthocyanins that reduce inflammation and promote neuron communication.

BE YOUR OWN COACH

Self assessment could be one of the most dynamic skills you can develop in your athletic journey. Learning to identify and understand your own fitness to perform and having the discipline to make the right choices, even when it's not ideal, sets you above the competition. You have to eliminate whatever is holding you back—make good changes! Success is a very stimulating positive reinforcement. ("What Is Mental Fitness?" 2021)

Demanding excellence from yourself can be daunting, but it can also be inspiring.

As you gain better command of your faculties, you'll find you can handle more workload, physically and mentally. Controlling reactions will keep you on top of the tasks you need to accomplish and eventually foster your capacity to handle more with increased ease and enjoyment.

A close cousin in reaction control is emotional control, or emotional management, for homeostasis. We thrive in consistency and routine. That doesn't mean you can't challenge yourself and your interactions, relationships, and dependencies. The results are not just sensational; our body reacts to emotional stimuli with chemicals that can cause harsh effects on our bodies, some very bad for our physical fitness and performance.

When you are in control of your emotions you can better choose how to change your behavior and attitude, and the better you feel… the better you feel! Chemical stability fosters mental fitness. ("Mental Fitness Explained by a CBT Psychologist" 2019)

FOUR PILLARS OF MENTAL FITNESS

The four established cornerstones of psychological wellness affect our decisions, behaviors, and actions. Think about how these apply to your game, your mood during play.

1. **Emotional self esteem** deals with our acceptance of ourselves and awareness about our internal landscape. Self confidence and reliance starts here.
2. **Social fitness** is how we interact, how we want to be perceived and how we think we are. This includes the realm of making friends, developing camaraderie, emotional ties, and partnership. Your ability to work with your team and trust comes from healthy social navigation.
3. **Financial fitness** concentrates on being in control of your life, not just wealth and money per se, but whether all of your needs are met or you are just surviving. Having time and the ability to have leisure and to turn leisure into a career like sports are all examples of financial fitness. This extends to training and being able to afford the means by which you gain your competitive skills.
4. **Physical fitness** has already been covered as being part of the whole. You need all of the above to reach optimal health and perform at a professional level.

("Four Pillars of Mental Fitness" 2019)

TRAINING YOUR BRAIN

Just like your body and your diet, you have ruts and ingrained habits you need to break. Reestablish new ones—better ones! You will have to realign these paths in the brain to make a new status quo, and changing your diet will have a huge impact on your transformation. The better foods you eat will help your brain just as much as they support your body. Enhancing your diet will enhance your ability to think and to act. Clarity of thought and pain-free motion will inevitably augment your cumulative improvement. The snowball effect is real.

Training your body and mind will lead to automatic responses. These autopilot responses are common, both good and bad. You have likely experienced many of them on the field or the court. Cultivating the right responses and programming your instincts starts with *muscle memory*. The idea of muscle memory means the whole system knows how to react on impulse correctly and automatically.

Quick thinking can be trained, raising your mental acuity. Reinforcing positive habits and goals with rewards and consistent repetition will hone your mind into a finely tuned instrument.

Similar to habitual conditioning, overpowering your limbic system's reflexes will give you the upper hand in your sport. When a ball comes flying at your head, without training and practice you might flinch or duck involuntarily. You can apply the disciplines from your training and dieting to cultivate these skills. Learn to respond, not react.

To feed the energy you need to cultivate an athletic mind, give it the nutrients it needs to rebuild and recover:

- Fatty acids in fish form a huge portion of the building blocks your brain needs to create nerve and brain cells. A large percentage of your brain is made of fat.

- Turmeric offers anti-inflammatory and antioxidant properties that have been linked to reducing depression. The key ingredient in turmeric is curcumin, a chemical which can actively enter the brain and interact, boosting the formation of new brain cells.
- Broccoli is full of Vitamin K which is responsible for generating dense fats in brain cells. (Jennings 2017)

SLEEP

Being in a present, mindful state requires mental acuity and sharpness that we can only get one way. Yes, food and activity play incredibly important roles, but none so much as the chemical process that is sleep. Sleep regulates the balance of the mind and regenerates our abilities to think and function properly.

Of course, it also provides the primary venue for healing and mending our muscles. Our sleep cycle is in fact cyclical. Good sleep equals a better head space, better body, which in turn helps you sleep better. Better sleep and the circle continues!

When you wake up refreshed, you feel compelled to go out and be productive. You might say you even feel a little competitive.

BRAIN FOOD

Several other foods are particularly good for your brain. Try incorporating some of these less common foods into your diet for stimulating your mental training alongside your physical routine.

- **Pumpkin seeds** for micronutrient minerals like magnesium, copper, and zinc.
- **Green tea** has a similar effect to coffee, but also contains the amino acid L-theanine that can cross the

blood-brain barrier directly. This promotes relaxation and relieves anxiety.
- **Nuts** support a healthy heart and give us Vitamin E that assists in memory and slowing mental decline. A healthier heart means a healthier brain!
- **Dark chocolate**, with a cocoa content of 70% or more, contains flavonoids that boost mood and mental sharpness.

COMPETITIVE NATURE

The instinct to compete and overcome is closely related to our willful drive to challenge our minds and develop our psychological and physiological prowess. We may be highly complex beings, but we are still essentially animals. The will to survive and thrive is built into us the same as any creature on the planet. With the added bonus of cognitive reasoning and creativity, the inevitable result translates competitiveness into *non-survival* outlets.

Competitiveness is functionally a two way street for our psyche. It is a natural drive within us in response to external conditions first and foremost, but indulging in our competitive side through positive activities generates good brain chemistry. From that nature we derive ambitiousness, as well as aspirations and hopes. When properly managed, successes and failures inspire us for even more pursuits and a determination to get back up and try again when we fall. ("Sport and Competition" 2019)

Despite our drives, we are also creatures of habit and routine. We can be prone to resist change and not want to learn. So we have to let our competitive nature take the lead to create new routines! Any coach will bench you or boot you if you aren't willing to take their advice or follow their expertise and guidance. Be your own coach, and don't let you make excuses.

As we train, our drive to win and make greater achievements

will grow. Winning will encourage that even more so! When you win, you want to keep winning, and you will want to raise the stakes and achieve those too!

That's naturally where competitive sports come in, because we want to be better, feel better, laugh more, and have more fun. We create games for that reason, first and foremost, before the desire to make a professional income doing what we love. After fun and enjoyment, it becomes personal achievement, raising the bar, aspirations for greatness, and an ongoing desire to make more of ourselves.

COMPETITIVE SPORTS

From the inspiration of our healthy impulses for fun and rivalry, sports have become one of our primary entertainment sources, both to view and participate. Indulging in pleasurable activities like watching your team win, brushing up on the stats from your favorite sport, or playing a round of hoops with your friends after work is very healthy and should be encouraged. Even reading this book for self improvement and leisure is an exercise in nurturing your abilities and fitness.

That's why they are called games to begin with, right? They are inherently supposed to be good for us, fun, challenging us to be better. Sports make you feel good, even when you lose!

Camaraderie and encouragement propel you forward. This is where teamwork comes from. Your peers challenge you and provide accountability to become better as you exchange skills and knowledge and share mutual successes. Sports instruct us how to teach and how to be taught. (Ives et al. 2020)

The added benefit of competing in a sport besides the obvious betterment of your health are the distractive elements that keep your fitness from feeling like a chore. Building the perfect athlete should be a serious task for you, but that does not mean that it cannot be fun and satisfying. You play your sport for a reason! Sports give us a destination to move toward with purpose, a trophy at the end of our accomplishments. Visualizing goals is far easier in the context of that framework.

Mentally focusing on one task at a time, and a task we want to be doing, starts us down the path to perfecting our craft. That's why you were able to pick up this book, to fill in another missing piece of your fitness puzzle. You're already on the right track, so keep it up and apply your focus to your diet, even if it is more abstract than shooting the ball or running drills. If it feels harder to control, that's your wayward mind trying to run away with your impulses. Hopefully, you can see why including sports in this chapter with mental health was intentional and necessary!

Confidence in yourself and your abilities got you to where you are. That process is ongoing and never ending. Nutrition is the tool you need to reach the next level of achievement. To adequately address the nutritional needs of each sport and their activities, take a look at the prominent fitness aspects associated with each one.

SPORT FOCUSES

Below is a handy list of the primary and auxiliary fitness components and which sports utilize them for reference in the next few sections of training and nutrition. As we begin to explore diets for the general attributes, you can correlate your sport to its needs and the suggested changes for that type. Please note, this includes most sports, but not all. There are dozens of variations on many of the fundamental sports, but the same skills apply. Take into account that most sports require all of the fitness categories in some capacity.

. . .

Endurance Focus Sports:

- Track and Field (Marathon, Hurdles, Sprints, Relays, Middle and Long Distances)
- Bicycling (Road Cycling)
- Soccer
- Basketball
- Tennis
- Dancing
- Volleyball
- Skiing (Cross Country)
- Boxing
- Squash
- Rowing
- Water Polo
- Field Hockey
- Rugby
- Lacrosse
- Swimming

Explosive Strength Focus:

- Sprinting (this applies across most sports in some capacity)
- Short Range Track and Field
- Volleyball
- Powerlifting
- Tennis
- Baseball
- Football

- Gymnastics (Vault, Uneven Bars, Still Rings, Horizontal Bar)

Flexibility Focus:

- Gymnastics
- Diving
- Wrestling
- Martial Arts (there are literally hundreds)
- Track and Field, Vaults, and Jumps
- Cheerleading
- Figure Skating
- Curling

Balance Focus:

- Equestrian Sports (Racing, Jumping, Dressage, Eventing)
- Ice Skating (Speed Skating, Hockey, Figure Skating, Synchronized Skating, Ice Dancing)
- Skiing (Downhill, Jumping)
- Gymnastics (Floor Exercise, Balance Beam, Pommel Horse, Parallel Bars)
- Rock Climbing (indoor and outdoor/natural)
- Golf
- Ballet
- Dancing (Competitive Dancesport)
- Snowboarding (Downhill, Jumping)
- BMX

- Mountain Biking
- Motocross
- Table Tennis
- Bowling
- Skateboarding

By now, you should have a very firm grasp of the fundamentals you need to move on, the meat and potatoes, if you will. The second half of this book is completely dedicated to your growth and planning your progress. In the next section, we will dive into the first stage of training and nutritional application, starting with beginners and working our way up to expert level incorporation of diet and micromanagement of your regimen. We'll even tell you all about diet plans that still let you eat delicious food while still meeting your goals!

PART THREE
BEGINNERS

CHAPTER 7
HOW YOU EAT

Take a breather, grab a glass of water and recover from your brain-workout. You've done an amazing job so far of keeping up as we've established the groundwork for your dietary adjustments. You made it through the preliminary information and are finally ready to get cooking!

Why don't we start with some appetizers? We'll look at how you go about making meals and your eating habits, then give you the basics on what to add and remove from your diet in the next chapter.

If you are already a pro, we promise we will work our way up to your so-called main courses, but for the beginner nutritionist, how you go about eating is just as important as what you eat. Methodology goes hand in hand with recipes.

COUNTING CALORIES

It's a catchy title to start with, but it is also a useful method! Counting your caloric intake is not the only method to lose or gain weight, but like we've touched on previously, *calories in/calories out* is a pretty safe baseline rule for most of your simple nutrition questions. You need to make certain you stay aware of how much you are eating no matter what level you reach. The higher you go, the more important each calorie's value, and where it came from, will be.

In regards to the whole topic of calorie consumption and keeping track of them, a better name to define the process would be *calorie management*. Calorie management more accurately sums up the fact that you need to be conscious of the nutritional value of the food you are eating, how much of it you can eat, and decisive about making the tough calls on what you are going to be putting, or more importantly not putting, in your body. Diet and nutrition boils down to calorie value, getting the most bang for your buck, and meeting your needs to get the returns you are aiming for by manipulating your meals. (Zelman 2009) There should be no variable that goes unchecked. Nothing in your food should be a mystery to you!

It may go without saying, but as we have been trying to relate, most of this process has to do with you taking control of your intake and closely accounting for every ounce of sustenance you consume. It's a big responsibility, but you owe it to yourself to be better.

More than likely, in order for you to do this, it will mean you will need to make the foods you eat, if you don't already, or at least carefully examine and research the locale where the prepared food you order comes from: its sourcing and how it is made. The crux of absolute control over your nutritional profile comes down to limiting unknowns and carefully documenting the details of your diet. For example, what is in the food you eat when you are eating at a restaurant? If you frequently go out to eat or get take out, you may not be able to analyze the foods you are supplying your athletic engine with.

Most restaurants can provide you with a list of nutritional charts for their menu items on request, or it might be available on their website. This may not include proprietary recipes or overly detailed ingredients, but it should give you a ballpark idea about what you're ingesting.

TIPPING THE SCALES

Maintaining mass– To maintain your muscle mass and overall body weight, you need to eat enough calories. Most of the effects of your total calorie count are cumulative over the week. If you eat a ton one day, and almost nothing the next, you won't experience a drastic change, other than feeling bad for not having eaten! In other words, meals can average out over short periods of time. Your body balance works in cycles, from sleep to digestion, and these cycles vary slightly for everyone. Even so, you won't likely gain much weight from a day of overeating, nor will you lose anything significant from starving yourself one day. Bloating, water retention, sodium levels, and other factors like temperature and how much you sweat will cause your weight to fluctuate throughout the week. When it comes down to actually gaining or losing mass, you have to commit to one type of intake over a period of time. The goal for stasis is to relatively eat an equal amount to the calories you burn over roughly a whole week cycle.

Losing mass– To lose weight, you need to lower the amount of calories you are eating. There is really no other way. Increasing your activity level significantly could outweigh your intake in rare cases, but cutting back on calories is much more effective and attainable.

In order to achieve weight loss, scientists estimate that a deficit of about 500 calories a day translates to about a pound of weight lost per week. That simply means you need to eat 500 calories less than you are burning. This is also a relatively safe figure for your health. You may be able to lose more, more quickly, but losing too much weight too rapidly, or gaining too much too swiftly is extremely hard on your body and can lead to many illnesses and problems. You want to make your body last, so don't put undue strain on it. ("Healthy Eating Plan" 2019)

Gaining mass– In order to add lean muscle mass, eat between 1.6-2.2 grams of protein per kilogram of bodyweight per day (0.75-1g protein/1 lb./day) The average healthy person can gain one to two pounds of lean muscle in a month.

Gaining weight purposefully should be done with the careful attention of your doctor and the right knowledge about your blood levels, vital statistics, and physiology. It is all too easy to start packing on the pounds without considering how it is affecting your blood pressure and cholesterol, or your hormonal balance. Consider trying to lean out and focus on cardiovascular fitness before aggressively tackling weight gains.

THE BURN

One of the most difficult parts of ascertaining your caloric needs is determining exactly how many you are burning, especially when you are trying to cut. Using the calorie counting method is a relative estimation that you can compare with common body-type models. Between this and your estimated BMI calculations, you can establish a fairly accurate activity level range and consult charts and common established norms for most body types similar to yours to get an idea.

Rules of 10 and 11– These rules of thumb are relative. According to this general model, men commonly burn 11 times their body weight in calories per day. For women, we multiply their weight by

10 for the same estimate. This figure is about as accurate as the food packaging label's 2000-calorie average for all people. Take that with a grain of salt and use this method only for approximating.

Simply count what you eat and keep the number lower than that estimate. That's pretty much the extent and equivalent of the home version. If you have access to professional equipment and personnel, you can actually figure out exactly how many calories you burn, how effective your diet and training plans are, as well as your efficiency at digesting individual nutrients. With the aid of modern medicine, you can find out a whole slew of other biological statistics that will perfect your school of athleticism. In many cases, discovering allergies or nutrient sensitivities reveals weaknesses you didn't know you were causing by eating foods unsuited to your biology. This is why examining everything you eat is so important for a baseline.

Without professional aid, you can alway order a handy little wrist gadget that can give you a close enough idea of what you are burning while in motion throughout the day and in your workout. Close enough to make sure you are not over eating, anyway.

CHANGING YOUR OUTLOOK

Another factor that controls, or at least contributes to our eating behaviors, is our culture and upbringing. We are conditioned to eat like our fellows, like our families, and like we are swayed by the media. Without getting too *talk about your feelings*, the psychology of eating has to be explored a bit as you aim to change things. One great example is no more of mom's rule to *clean your plate*. We get it, she wants you to grow big and strong and not waste food. But you are big and strong now, and you should only eat what you need.

By now, we know food interacts with how we feel. In addition to memory based favorites and nostalgia programming, this reaction to food can largely be blamed on the production of serotonin that regulates sleep and mood which takes place mostly in the gastrointestinal tract. 95% of your serotonin comes from your intestines! So your guts literally control your mood. No wonder you get cranky when you're hungry.

Good food makes us feel good, but that's a loaded statement. Good is subjective to taste. Delicious treats activate the happy chemicals in your brain, including the foods that hold little or no nutritional value for you. Modifying your diet with healthy food will make you feel good physically in more ways than one, and for longer. Retraining your mind to crave better foods and your body to rely and demand healthier foods is part of the ongoing process. You will become less dependent on the sensations your crutch foods give you as you fill nutritional voids in your diet. Besides, these dependencies are holding you back from athletic perfection!

Don't worry, you can still have them occasionally as a reward. They just can't be the norm.

As you can see, our behaviors define a lot of our diet. Think about the habits you have around eating and how they affect your daily routine and your exercise program. Your schedule and many other external influences alter the course of your mealtimes, forcing convenience to supersede quality of nutrition. Grabbing a burger and fries on your way home from work is easy. Planned meal preparation would have a healthy, balanced dinner waiting for you at home in the fridge.

Of course, the first step is recognizing the problem and having the desire for change. Discipline rears its head again. Take a close look at your tendencies and compulsions and what drives those behaviors. What can you remove from the equation to stop the cycle?

Do you always eat poorly at a certain place, or a certain time, or under specific conditions? These are all good things to know. This is how you head off your bad habits and make way for new ones. What are the times you want to eat in contrast to when you actually do? Are you always tempted to eat late at night?

Sorry in advance if we are getting a little 'Food Guru' on you, but positivity and negativity have drastic effects on your brain and mood. Your attitude can be the difference between success and failure. In order to make your life easier in the process, consistency is key. Don't expect to change overnight. That goes for every aspect from the inside out. You won't suddenly become a disciplined person if you aren't—change takes time. This is why we are addressing the issue as one entire project.

TIPS AND TECHNIQUES

Sometimes the problem in a structure is a lack of solid foundational skills. Here are some proper eating techniques to help you implement better habits by eating correctly. These techniques may seem simple, but they work as well for the weekend hobby bicyclist as they do for the Olympic swimmer:

- Slower eating. Chew your food. Enjoy it. Savor it.
- Increase your water intake, especially right before a meal. Drinking more water serves multiple purposes. It not only fills you part of the way up, it also primes your gut for digestion and helps you absorb the useful nutrients in your food. Have we mentioned how good water is for you?
- Stop when you're full, you don't need the extra insulin response to drag you down. Overeating is hard on your digestive tract and your body in general.
- If you can work it into your schedule, cook your own food. You will become more conscious of what you

- make yourself. This will help your financial budget as well as your calorie budget.
- Be present when you eat. Pay attention to the act of eating because absent snacking is the gain killer!
- Don't shop for groceries without a list! Always plan ahead and outline your meals. Once you have the good stuff at home, you will be more inclined to use it and follow your regimen.
- Eating less just before bed is recommended for better sleep. You don't need all that food sitting in your stomach all night. (West 2019)

OVER INDULGENCE

Let's be honest, we know when we do this! But the concept in general is simple: moderation. Use a little less sauce, dressing, etc. One facet we will explore here is still enjoying your food, and the allowance for cheats at every level of fitness and strictness.

On the other hand, this does mean you need to cut down or cut out calorie heavy beverages. Sodas and beers are extremely calorie dense, and drinking your calories will not only put you over your daily caloric allotment, but also leave you feeling sluggish and still hungry in both the short and long run.

Sugar is not your friend, unfortunately. It has its place. But ways to manage your use of it can help you trim out unnecessary and ineffective calories. Try to take your tea or coffee without it or just use less. By the same token, you usually know which food you really shouldn't eat. Start listening to your inner athlete.

TAKING A CLOSER LOOK

In recent years, new focal fields of study are emerging all the time as our research of food and humanity grows. With more resources and specialists on the task, understanding our relationship with our bodies gets a little easier every year. Like we mentioned in a previous chapter, nutritional sciences are relatively young, but we are extremely fortunate to be alive during the exponential advancement of those sciences.

One of these emergent schools of study is Nutrition Psychology which investigates the inextricable interdependency of food, body, and mind. Moreover, science is examining how our relationship with food plays into our social interactions, dictates our behavior, and determines our own culinary practices. (Cleveland Clinic 2016)

From the converging specialties of so many other medical and scientific fields, nutritional psychology has developed the DMHR (Diet-Mental Health Relationship) model that aims to uncover lies in our diet we have come to believe for many reasons. We all know there are chemicals in many of the foods we eat that lead to mental distress and neurological and psychological disorders as well as physical ailments. With the help of new research, we can begin to eliminate them. The issue is massive and far reaching, but take this to heart as an incentive to be more interested where you source your food from to avoid as many toxic additives as possible. (Psychology, Nutritional 2022)

Studies show that changing your diet can add years to your life, in addition to the short term benefits. Dietary risk factors in western diets are mostly due to elevated quantities of processed and preservative infused foods. (Brown 2022) Nutritional voids are another issue that many other countries fill naturally with spices and simpler, naturally grown foods due to availability and less chemical modification.

MAKING MOVES

Think about what you do and what you want to do. What is your primary athletic outlet and focus and how can what you eat support the demands of your sport? With the knowledge you have so far, you should be able to start wrapping your head around it. How can your diet plans get you where you want to be? Do you need to be lighter, heavier, stronger, or more endurant? The goal is the first step.

It can feel like you are taking away all of the things you love, but it's not true! Sometimes, it takes a little coaxing and tricking our brains into doing the right thing.

Tricks to supplementing your diet instead of *losing* things:

- You can always eat more vegetables. They are filling and good for you, and almost always low in calories. This can help you start to control your calorie profile while staying full.
- Switch to the raw ingredient. If you always buy instant rice or oatmeal, try picking up the dry ingredient and taking the time to cook it. It's not that much longer or harder!
- As you increase your activity level, increase your protein intake. Lean protein only!
- Cook things in equally delicious but different ways. Roast your vegetables and meats instead of frying them. (Bjarnadottir 2017)

When it comes to sweets, divide them out into small, limited portions to prevent over indulgence. Don't just grab the bag! Cutting deserts out cold turkey is not only hard on your willpower, but can be rough on your system if you are used to getting sugar regularly. Weaning off of sweets will allow your body to adjust.

FOOD DIARY/JOURNAL

The final nutritional tool that you must begin immediately is a food diary. Keeping track of your meals and calories will serve so many purposes. Simply being aware of everything you put in your body keeps you attentive and makes you more discerning. No more out of sight, out of mind! Writing out your plan and your actions works to cement new behaviors and will also increase memory capacity and acuity through activity.

Tracking your nutrients, calories, and supplements will lead to you narrowing in on what you need. Why do I feel this way = what did I eat? The answers will present themselves through careful notation and calculation. (Institute of Medicine 2012)

Your food diary will also serve to lay out your schedule and can be combined with a workout journal of your routine and your benchmarks and achievements. Not only will this provide accountability, but it will make you become extremely consistent. Our bodies respond very well to patterns, and you will enhance your gains immensely by sticking to a tight program.

All of your planning and laying down a clear path for groundwork will limit deviation from subsequent goals.

This is how champion athletes behave, and you are on your way to becoming just that.

CHAPTER 8
EATING FIT

Now that you have started your food diary to keep track of all of your snacks and pre-game fueling, use that new tool to plan your week. Recording what you do after the fact is all fine and good, but forethought is even more tactical to reach your destination. As you begin to understand how many calories you are burning in your exercise regimen and your average daily burn, you can cater your cooking to accommodate.

MEAL PLANNING

Athletes often complain about a lack of flavor and variety in their diets. Unfortunately, for convenience and when you are doing a lot of the prep work, it is easier to make a bunch of the same thing ready for fast fuel. However, you don't have to eat bland boiled chicken, vegetables, and rice for every meal.

Not all of us are Michelin chefs, so getting creative with your meals can be a bit of a chore. Be sure and use all the resources at your disposal. There are unlimited websites and cookbooks out there for ideas that cater to conscious nutrition.

Most importantly, as you begin to sculpt your ideal diet, keeping foods you like for sanity will help you stay the course.

Nevertheless, you will need to make a few hard calls on what you can no longer eat.

PROCESS OF ELIMINATION

We all have our cheat treats. There is really nothing wrong with it! Unless you are cheating and eating them constantly. Then they are no longer treats, this is just your diet.

A University of Michigan study recently observed the life-potential in over 5,800 foods to weigh their value for and against your health. For example, a hot dog has a relative life cost of about 36 minutes of poorer health. The study was conducted to show how better foods gain you a better life. Higher quality foods make you feel better and live longer. ("Small Changes in Diet" 2021)

In other words, while your body is digesting and processing bad stuff, your health and life quality are lower for having ingested something of poor nutrition. Even once you recover and eliminate the waste of that meal, your body suffers for it. Keep that idea in mind when you choose your food.

Simple eliminations/limitations can trim down the unnecessary elements from your diet to make definitive changes:

- **Sodas and beers**– As sad as this seems, both are high in calories and sugars, not to mention the alcohol that is never good for athletic performance. If you do decide to indulge in a drink to take the edge off, maybe try a liquor based drink with a no sugar mixer for a fun night. Unfortunately, diet sodas are not much better. The chemical sweeteners used to simulate sweetness have very negative effects on your brain and are not great for your body. In place of sodas try unsweetened teas or low calorie water flavoring if you just have to drink a flavored beverage.

- **Juice and juice cocktails–** Unless you are squeezing the juice right from the fruit, it's probably a good idea to leave these products on the shelf or limit your intake. Even the fresh squeezed variety has almost as much sugar as a soda, even if it is marginally better for you. Additionally, the argument that it's fruit falls flat without any of the fiber or essential elements left behind in the flesh of the fruit you juiced. Once again, moderation is key.
- **Fried chips and other fried foods–** There are other snacks! Baked chips are a bit better even if they still contain large amounts of bad oils and fats. Try popcorn with just a bit of olive oil and salt!
- **Salad dressing and rich sauces on meat and sides–** We all love rich flavors, but most sauces and dressings are chock full of sugar, unhealthy oils, and preservatives. Experiment with making your own dressings for salad with olive oil, vinegar, and seasonings, with dijon mustard or a dash of honey to thicken.
- **Seasoning is fine–** You don't have to eliminate flavor! Just be conscious of how much salt you are adding. If you are highly active and drink plenty of water it's likely not an issue, but if you suffer from any blood pressure problems be mindful.
- **Lowering sugar–** We already addressed the sugary drinks, but this goes for a majority of sugar heavy products. One of the other concerns with sweet delicacies is that they also tend to be loaded with full fat butter and other rich dairy items. When you do enjoy a pastry or pie at least carefully take the time to choose which sugary treat you will have. Even better,

make the desert yourself with a meaningfully chosen, lower sugar recipe.
- **Saturated fats, butters and spreads–** The oils in butter replacements are not all good for you due to the need to simulate texture and flavor. Sometimes the alternative product is worse for you than the original!
- **Dairy–** Not all of it! Just the full fat items that contain a lot of lactose. Milk is actually full of sugar, believe it or not! That's why it has so many calories. Read your labels, especially where dairy and dairy alternatives are concerned. Dairy also has inflammatory effects on most people, so consider if keeping it in your diet is worth it in the long run or if you could live without it.
- **Breakfast cereals–** There's not many of them that are good for you! A sugar rush to start your day is not recommended. A few, like bran flakes (without frosting), and some other wholegrain-based, high-fiber cereals exist on the market. Just be cautious about the added sugar content and advertised supplements like "high protein." This often includes the milk you would add.
- **Red meats–** Consume less red and particularly processed, hormonally modified meats.

ALL PART OF A BALANCED DIET

There has been much debate over what the ideal percentage each of the macronutrients should play in the average diet. Early on in the study of food science, much of the prescribed data was based on some fairly notable biases. As an example, the promotion of wheat in the North American diet primarily spawned out of the 1940s war times and the need to feed the masses. This added to the subsidization of certain crops over others that yielded faster, more bountiful harvests and weighed heavily on the focal foods that people needed to be eating for a healthy lifestyle. Not to say that wheat and corn are in any way bad foods. They have their place in a well-rounded diet.

Since then, there has been a lot of research and discovery that has led to reform and a more accurate message about nutrition and diet from governmental nutritional education. Current percentage suggestions according to the USDA (United States Department of Agriculture):

- 45-65% from carbohydrates
- 10-35% from proteins
- 20-35% from fats

("How to Determine the Best" 2016)

This is not wrong, per se. The average person could function on this layout very successfully. And frankly, most people eat far more carbs in their diet than that daily recommended percentage, which is not ideal. Most folks don't get nearly enough protein in their diet. So if anyone relied on this model, or increased their protein intake based on it, it would probably do them a lot of good.

But these aren't athletes we're talking about. You are!

Ratios are useful, but they have been shown to have little effect on weight loss diets as long as the dieter is eating a deficit of calories. On the other hand, when training and moving into athleticism, ratios will become much more important for meeting your needs. For now, we can disregard percentages and ratios and focus instead on the main groups of foods.

- Grains
- Vegetables
- Fruits
- Low fat dairy

- Lean protein
- Nuts
- Water (However much you are drinking, you likely could increase it.)

You should eat some or all of these items in your diet at any level of athleticism, and, of course, some more than others depending on your athletic needs down the line. We will break that down more in depth as we move into intermediate and advanced athletic nutrition in the next sections.

By consuming foods from each of these groups you raise your likelihood of receiving all of the nutrients you need to grow. As we get more and more complex, you can start to identify specifics within each category you prefer and need to focus on in your regimen.

DINING IN STYLE

Several factors come to mind when approaching your choice in diet plans. A multitude of online resources exist to help you, as always, but you must take into consideration what works for you not only in body, but in life.

Many styles of diets are very effective and sound appealing until you attempt to apply them to your everyday life. Observe the requirements of a diet plan for these elements:

- **Accessibility–** Can you get the foods suggested? Are there alternatives in your area that make it possible?
- **Sustainability–** Is it something you think you can manage and continue?
- **Budget–** Can you afford this diet?
- **Owning it–** Can you adapt the precepts of the plan and make it your own? As you gain experience you'll find

that you only need a framework offered by an expert to insert your own favorites and cornerstones. ("Weight Loss Diet Plans" 2021)

Once you ascertain if the diet is manageable for you, start it! In a few weeks you should see if the results are beginning to meet your expectations if you stick with it. You can also tweak and adjust parts of it that don't suit you in practice.

You will come across so many styles of diets as you establish your program. A few of these have excellent aspects that you can incorporate into your plan.

Intermittent fasting– This diet revolves around your sleep fasting for a long period without food. This diet limits calorie intake by shortening the time frame you can eat in. Hunger has been shown in some studies to foster increased calorie burn in the short run. The danger of this diet is mitigating the threshold when you start entering starvation. On the plus side, fasting resets insulin sensitivities, can assist in hormonal production and balance, and reduce inflammation from roller coaster cycles of digestion.

Veggie based diets– Vegetarianism is an option, but not a must for most people. If you decide to highlight vegetables as the primary source of your nutritive intake, just make sure you are eating enough protein. Vegetarians often suffer from a lack of certain nutrients by omitting meat and animal products. You need plenty of protein and iron for training.

Lower carb or no carb– These diets reduce or minimize your carb intake by either cutting down on your common carbohydrates or exchanging simple starches and over-processed foods for natural high fiber raw ingredients and whole grains. Be very skeptical of zero carb diets, as they exclude most vegetables and starches. Overly specific diets can lead to deficiencies.

Paleo– The paleo mentality cuts out most processed foods primarily. That's not a bad thing. This nutritional ideology is focused around a natural diet, which has been shown to lower cholesterol and high blood pressure. Its shortcomings show a limitation by excluding some useful food groups like legumes and some good dairy from your options.

All of these diets have their benefits and detriments that can be avoided with planning and modification. No diet is perfect for everyone, so you will need to fine tune whatever program you choose. (Raman 2019)

MISSING OUT

The most pressing issue for most people are the missing pieces of their dietary profile. There is inevitably something you are not eating that you should be. If you struggle with overeating starches and not eating enough veggies, make vegetables the main course and eat them first. You'll have less room for starches and sugars once you're done.

Additions that many people lack in their regular diet:

- **Greek yogurt–** Excellent protein. Digestive cultures.
- **Nuts, legumes–** Tons of protein, fats, and minerals.
- **Dark greens–** Micronutrients galore. Many also have

very healthy carbs and other chemicals that promote clean blood.
- **Eggs–** Great, nearly pure protein, good fats, and good cholesterol.
- **Vitamin supplements–** If you aren't already taking them. Look at what is in them, and what your body type typically needs. Things like low iron and low calcium can make you feel terrible and you have never been able to figure out why.
- **Vitamin D–** Supports hormone production, muscle growth, and sleep. Most people do not get enough sunlight for their body to naturally produce enough.
- **Popcorn–** Such a good snack! Popcorn is an excellent source of fiber and much lower in calories than chips (as long as it's not smothered in butter or oil).
- **Coconut, avocado and olive oil–** Use instead of canola, vegetable, or sunflower oils.
- **Fiber–** Analyze how much you are getting and look at how to increase it. It will regulate your blood sugar spikes and keep you fuller longer and make you want to eat less.

Remember those essential micronutrient minerals? Here are the ones you don't produce that you need to add through food and where you can find them: (Harvard Health Publishing 2016)

- **Zinc–** Shellfish, beef, lamb , pork, legumes, seeds, nuts
- **Magnesium–** Dark chocolate, avocados, tofu, legumes, nuts
- **Vitamin C–** Bell peppers, citrus fruits, broccoli, cauliflower, tomatoes
- **Vitamin E–** Sunflower seeds, almonds, red bell pepper, mango, asparagus, avocado

(West 2018; Franziska 2018; Harvard School of Public Health 2012; Harvard 2012)

There are innumerable diets out there, and we cannot cover them all here. Your main focus should be on finding one that suits your desired outcome and needs. Find foods you like within the spectrum of macronutrients to help you fill in the gaps in your diet.

Online resources like the Mayo Clinic and Mercer Health have available diet plans and health surveys to help you establish where you are at in your diet, activity level, and needs. Be wary of fad diets in magazines and media. Many are well researched and sound, but the source and author might not convey risks that come with certain aspects or deficiencies in their program. Plans from certified dieticians and doctors are a much safer bet.

CHAPTER 9
GETTING ACTIVE

Now that you have begun to shift your thinking and your approach to eating, we have to look at getting active to maximize your results. Your best athletic accomplishments begin with the synergy of diet and action. If you are already involved in a program of exercise, take this section as a refresher course and see if there are any fundamentals you are lacking in your approach. Fitness is a never-ending circuit of discovery and enhancement.

PROOF IN THE PUDDING

While it may seem daunting to tackle both halves of the issue of nutrition and exercise, scientists from the University of Michigan have recently shown that better results are achieved both mentally and physically when you work on both facets simultaneously. In their study, subjects who only managed to work on one or the other showed significantly less progress than the group that changed both their diet and exercise routines. Change is hard regardless, so you may as well get it over with, right? The sooner you get started, the sooner you will see results!

The same goes for the beginner enthusiast or the expert athlete. You must constantly review and refine your methods of perfecting your athleticism. If you have been hesitating on making those subtle changes to your routine because of laziness, or staying in your comfort zone, now is the time to get on it! Wherever you find yourself in your progress, there is always something new to add, a new goal to strive for.

So let's talk about making moves and exercising more. Whether that means literally getting out and running more frequently or moving more weight, faster and harder. More is how you move forward!

While you may see some changes over the first few weeks, true, long-lasting changes take time. Sticking with a diet and a workout plan for the long haul is the only way to make lasting changes. Unfortunately, subtle changes are even harder, but so much more satisfying. It's a lot like figuring out a little tweak on your golf swing that suddenly makes your drive much more powerful. You'll wonder why you never figured it out before!

Your body works in roughly 12 week cycles so expect to spend around 90 days doing the work before the real big stuff settles in. Some of the progress will come in swells after the initial trial period, and that's when you will really need to ride that wave of positivity and success.

CAPABILITY

This not only includes your physical prowess but your free time, work schedule, and other responsibilities in relation to your work out.

Experts recommend doing 150 minutes of aerobic activity per week. Anything over that is even better. This basically translates to at least working out in some capacity at least three days a week. For beginners anything over five days could be an excess. You can determine what level you find yourself at.

There are a number of factors that play into how often you

work out or train early on in your fitness journey. The first is how long you have been working out. Your *fitness age*. This is the cumulative experience your body has at doing exercise.

Alongside that experience, you should be aware of your max heart rate, your general conditioning, and your overall strength levels in training. See a doctor to note things like blood pressure and resting heart rate, along with conditions you should be aware of to caution or temper your training. Often, this doesn't exclude you completely from an activity, but it may require you taking the time to warm up and find a sustainable pulse. An introductory circuit may be necessary to work through and bolster your faculties before moving on to a more intense regimen.

With experience comes knowledge and skill. What you are used to doing, have done in the past, and can once again acclimate to are all admissible to populating the exercises in your current processes. Also, take into consideration what you like to do, your favorite exercises and sports, and what you need to work on to accommodate them.

At the end of the day, setting realistic goals and committing to what you can reasonably manage will start meaningful progress toward any improvement. Just like this book!

MAKING A ROUTINE

Careful regimentation and outlining set the pace for every workout. Have a plan going in and do not deviate from it. So much time is wasted in gyms deciding what to do next, and even more at home when you have ample distractions. You need a game plan! If you arrive with a road map you will never slow down, and the momentum can help you keep your energy up.

Focus and intention are your biggest mental allies in the gym —whether at home or at a club. You are there to get work done! Be present and acknowledge each move you are doing, focusing on the muscle-mind connection.

Finding the right recipe for your success is important. If you need to work out at home to avoid the distractions of socializing at the gym, then do that. Or, if that doesn't work and you find yourself being lazy at home, go somewhere to work out. Even if it's not a gym and it's running at the park, fine! Training can be done anywhere. Find what motivates you and keeps you moving!

Results won't happen overnight. This means you need to give your chosen work out a chance to work before you move on to the next thing. And if it's hard or uncomfortable, maybe it's exactly what you should be doing. Don't flit from one thing to the next or you will never see any real progress. You know what dedication looks like. That's why we're here.

THE SPLIT

Deciding on a workout plan can be tricky. You can construct your own if you feel confident enough in your physical fitness know-how, or seek out good sources of reputable routines to try and see what suits you. There are endless options online and in books and magazines of great athletes who have done it all before and share their methods. Many of them are tried and true, so you can't go wrong sticking with the classics. Anything in a routine that you cannot perform or you feel unsure about—don't do! Make it your own.

Stick with it! Sometimes you have to change routines because it is just not a good fit in your current state, but ask yourself if you are stopping because you can't do it, you don't like it, or you just don't want to! Sometimes, doing the things we don't want to do most is exactly what we should do. Acknowledging a weak point, addressing it, and fixing the problem is exactly in line with what we are doing in this book. Better ingredients make better food. The food in this case is your body. The ingredients are the workouts—in case you didn't catch the analogy.

Speaking of analogies, this brings us to a bit more of a metaphorical look at balance, in how we manage our schedules, work, fun and family. Keeping all of the balls in the air at once is difficult and requires a set of skills and training all its own. Making changes to this system can be upsetting, and you will need to practice balance more than ever to make progress.

Training your balancing mastery will also help you manage your regimen, your diet, and implement them effectively while keeping your other responsibilities in check. Use your food diary. Make lists. Execute them!

This is the part of the book where we have to emphasize that nutrition isn't just about food and exercise. Food is your life. Life is also your sport.

CHECKMARKS

Taking measurements is a great tool for progress. While your weight is very subjective to your actual fat content and muscle mass, the numbers can track progress more easily than a blood panel work up. Measuring your circumferences at different points on your body lets you keep track of your starting point on a cycle and how you grow. Setting milestones of gains and losses visually is a great way to motivate you. Seeing real results always reinforces better behavior and incentivizes you to continue with the work.

Weigh and measure yourself at regular intervals for encouragement and tracking:

- **BMI–** The body mass index—a value obtained from a person's mass and height.
- **Scale weight–** (If you have a scale with a BIA or BIS feature it can give you an additional body-fat estimate.)

- **Measurements**– At the peak of the bicep, thigh, chest (across nipples), waist, and belly.
- **Times and reps**– More important than your physical appearance are your gains. Track your repetitions and weight capacity in your resistance training and your time and pace when doing cardiovascular exercises. This is your real progress!

Try to remember that weight is a only number and should only be used as a guideline (Until you are moving into professional levels where each ounce of body weight matters for weight class, mobility, and extreme body fat content control). That is why knowing your body and its tendencies is crucial to have reasonable expectations and make reasonable progress. This doesn't mean you can't reach your target athleticism, but rather helps you garner better understanding on how to get there. You may surprise yourself.

SPLITS AND FREQUENCY

Depending on how you divide your workout can change how often you need to do it. You don't want to overwork any muscle group. If you are working on a power split, you may only focus on one muscle group per week. Volume training spreads the work for every muscle group across the week to avoid soreness and achieve a greater workload cumulatively. HIIT (High Intensity Interval Training) workouts use bursts of intense output in cycles.

If you are *young* in your fitness age, you can easily become too sore and set yourself back with days of recovery. Limit what you do to what you can, and then work up from there. Any athlete would take this sound advice for making advances in their craft.

Starting with a full body and compound exercise plan is the best way to build a foundation of fitness. Working in some isolation exercises will accentuate auxiliary muscles and mix up your sets. Everyone loves how they feel and look doing certain exercises. Use that to get psyched!

Doing a simple full body circuit three days a week starts you off. After four to six weeks, look at switching it up to a more diverse plan that adds a day or two and divides your muscle groups up. At this stage, you should try to hit each group twice a week for durability and endurance. Anything more than five days a week should be carefully considered. You could fatigue or cause yourself injury if you aren't accustomed to the workload.

Assess your goals at the start of your new cycle and decide what is best for your ideal results. In what way are you out of shape? Should you do a phase of compensating cardio to get your endurance where it needs to be before starting a high repetition, high intensity routine? Take the journey in stages. You wouldn't jump straight into power cleans without working on your shoulder press and deadlifts first.

Alongside frequency, you have to incorporate and balance intensity. Push too hard, you will be too sore to work out again soon, or you could injure yourself. Too little, and you won't make any progress. Finding that sweet spot can free up your weekly layout. More intensity could liberate a day, lowering it could spread the split over more days, but shorter workouts.

WARMING UP

Lubricating your joints and priming your muscles with blood will ensure a powerful and successful workout.

Cardiovascular Exercises

Getting outside if you can is just good for you—mind and body. Even better than just long form running, marathoners train by cycling, walking, and running in increments and adjust them for intensity and challenge. Try doing a 15-30 minute walk/run, running/jogging for 30 seconds and walking for one and a half minutes between each run.

Solid state cardio is good for you, especially to build endurance and cardiovascular function, but keeping your body at a mid-level heart rate and temp for a long period of time is not as effective as interval conditioning for burning calories or putting your body in a state of work that it will need to grow.

Resistance can be just as intense if done with cardio intensity and high repetition.

Aerobics classes help with exterior motivation and get your heart rate up for a set time.

Strengthening Exercises

- Weight training and heavy resistance
- Explosive movements, fast-twitch routines, sprints
- Volume training for balanced maintenance and less muscle recovery

Hypertrophy and Recovery

- Stretching
- Meditation and yoga can help you get a handle on your mind game
- 150 minutes/week of hard activity will increase blood flow, help sleep, heart and lung health
- Sleep and food

SAMPLE SPLITS:

<u>MWF</u>

- 10 minutes warm up—jumping jacks—jog
- 30 minutes full body circuit of compound exercises—push ups—squats— pulldowns/pullups—deadlifts
- 15 minutes interval cardio walk/run
- 15 cool down stretch

<u>MTWTh</u>

- 10 minutes dynamic warm up and stretch

<u>M/W</u>
Alternating push upper and lower—squats/push ups or bench—variations

<u>T/Th</u>
Alternating sets pull upper and lower—lunges/rows—variations

- 10 minutes high intensity interval cardio-burpees
- 10 minutes cooldown stretches

You get the idea. Make sure you are drinking plenty of water throughout your workout and eat a high protein meal shortly after with some sugars and fats to assist in nutrient uptake and cell replenishment. Sports drinks can replace lost electrolyte salts, but be careful with the sugar content.

Consider bringing a friend along. Working with a partner will help you keep with the activity as you hold each other accountable, and it makes the experience more fun. Challenge each other! It is also safer to have someone there in case of injuries, especially if you do something with a margin of danger like heavier lifting or bicycling away from cities, hiking, etc.

GET THE BALL ROLLING

Aside from gym training and fundamentals like running, getting active or diversifying your athletic portfolio can be very fulfilling and help you make strides in your career. If you already have a sport you love, try to do it more often—hone your craft. Be open to trying new athletic activities as well. Challenge amplifies your skills. As you do this, begin to look at what you need to enhance your body to improve at each sport or hobby.

Common sports that can easily become more than a hobby:

- Jogging
- Weight lifting
- Bicycling
- Fishing
- Golf
- Soccer
- Basketball
- Boxing
- Swimming
- Rock Climbing

PART FOUR
INTERMEDIATE

CHAPTER 10
COOKING SMART

At the intermediate level of athleticism you should start becoming more energy efficient as well as a competent exerciser. Your moderate *athletic age* puts you in a perfect spot to start incorporating pro-level advice and influence with enough wherewithal to avoid injury and beginner's mistakes.

To become like the best, taking tips and staples from what they do is a wise place to start. No, you shouldn't adopt an Olympic runner's routine off the bat. That level takes years to reach, and every routine is all encompassing. If you aren't training four to six hours a day in your sport, you don't need to eat like you are. So we will just take away the meaning behind how pro athletes eat and work, and apply it to the steps leading there, or to whatever final level your athletic path is taking you.

BREAKING THE FAST

First off, breakfast is imperative. Certain special diets withstanding, if you want to eat like a pro, you must eat your breakfast. This meal sets the stage for the whole day. Especially if you wake and exercise soon after, you are coming off of a long stint with no food. Some trainers advocate fasting and working out prior to eating, and there is some evidence to show for it. However, this is case by case, and just like most things athletically related, it is not suitable for every person. Your body needs fuel to work, and you cannot afford to crash in the middle of your workout, or worse in competition. Not to mention the rippling effect that can hinder your performance at your job. ("Exercise and Eating Healthy" 2014)

That brings us to a very important trifecta that comes straight from the top. Successful athletes all have three things in common: balance, variety, and moderation. The first is most important to apply to all aspects of your life. You won't make any progress if you are stretched too thin in any area. Balance your meals, your free time, your work, your exercise, and your sleep. Variety ties in closely to make sure you get enough mental stimulation, rest, productivity, and all of the nutrients your body needs while not overexerting yourself. Finally, moderation tempers the other two by keeping a keen eye on when to pause, and analyzing what is working and what isn't. ("Nutrition and Physical Activity" 2020)

Every ingredient is as important as the next when you are trying to make the perfect dish. While this book is not designed as a recipe book on how to make delicious and savory cuisine, it is the recipe for a methodology to apply over your entire athletic life.

PROBLEM SOLVING

Unfortunately, there are always more hurdles to address in nutrition. Here are a few intermediate tips on how to keep refining your eating habits.

- **Skipping meals**– Missing meals causes big disruptions in your systems.
- **Undereating**– There is a fine line between dieting and starving yourself. Even when you cut down on calories, you still need to meet certain nutritional quotas to

function. Besides, starvation leads to overeating on the back end, which defeats the purpose of trying to cut calories.
- **Fasting**– Fasting is another thing altogether. This practice should only be attempted with careful supervision and consultation with your doctor.
- **Overeating**– All too easy to do nowadays. Even as an athlete, you may be overshooting how much you really need, or how intense you think your activity level is. (Ron 1995)

Bad habits are just that—bad! You probably already know what behaviors you need to purge from this list. Dissect your diet, your training process, and regimen and find your weaknesses. Systematically phase them out and establish new norms.

MAKING DEMANDS

As you inevitably increase your workload, both in volume and intensity, your caloric needs will also grow. Taking a sharp look at input/output and tracking those numbers demands closer attention alongside your athletic growth.

Familiarizing yourself with guidelines of brackets of activity will better formulate your culinary compensation. A good bracket breakdown according to the health department of Victoria, Australia outlines:

- **Low intensity** = 30 minutes/day ~150-300 calories
- **Medium intensity** = 60 minutes/day ~350-475 calories
- **Endurance** = 1-3 hours/day ~500-725 calories
- **Extreme endurance** = 4+ hours/day ~750-950 calories

("Calories Burned During Fitness" 2017)

Now, the amount of calories you burn during those time frames varies greatly based on the difficulty of the exercises you're doing, your body mass, fitness level, sex, and body type. You can burn anywhere from 300 calories doing an hour of moderate walking to burning almost 1,000 calories running strenuously. These figures are rough estimates to give you a ballpark. Besides that, by now you should have a pretty good idea of your numbers. And remember, you also burn calories throughout the day in addition to your workout.

Regardless of the exact number, it is highly recommended that during longer workouts you should consume 50-100 calories every half hour after the first 90 minutes to maintain muscle function and performance.

In terms of what this means for your food, you already know that you need to eat enough to keep up with your schedule. The difference as you start to become a seasoned athlete is to change your ratios to meet the needs of your activity.

Prescribed percentages for intermediate athletes:

- 55-60% carbohydrates
- 15-20% proteins
- 20-30% fats

The variance accounts for your specific sport, but during an era of growth and acceleration you will need a lot of carbohydrates and fats, even more than protein, to support energy demands, cell growth, and hormonal production. Your muscle will almost take care of itself as long as you are providing it with adequate protein.

WINS AND LOSSES

Outside of the calorie matching of maintaining your weight, at this stage you are likely settling on some of the specific goals you want to reach in regards to your physique. It is so very important to make sure you do not gain or lose weight too quickly for long lasting and healthy results.

It is possible to safely lose fat while retaining your muscle mass, at a rate between a half pound to two pounds, if you are carefully monitoring your nutrient base. Losing weight too fast inevitably leads to muscle loss as well. Cutting is hard, but you can manage it if you are patient.

During weight loss, there is a much higher risk of dehydration as you lose a lot of water when burning fat stores. Keep your water intake consistent and plentiful.

Gaining muscle takes even longer, so be prepared for the long haul. Steady muscle growth tops out around two pounds per month. Upkeep of muscle fiber requires 1-1.5 gram of protein per kilogram of bodyweight in athletes (.45-.70 grams of protein per pound). More can be eaten during the gain phase, approaching 2-2.5 grams per kilo (~ 1-1.25 grams per pound). Anything over this can be taxing on your kidneys as excess protein is excreted primarily in urine.

Like we've mentioned before, you do not want to make long or short term adjustments to your body in the event season or near competition. The off-season is for making changes to your system. When it comes time for performance, your main purpose should be upkeep.

If you have not carefully monitored your weight, BMI, and your measurements, now is the time to begin. Following any peaks and valleys will become more and more crucial as you reach professional echelons of performance. Any drastic consistency shifts in your body could be a sign of trouble.

MACRO-MASTER

For your greater intents and purposes, carbs should now make up more than half of your daily caloric intake. Studies show that 60-70% of energy used in exercise comes from carbs in the bloodstream followed by retained stores in muscle tissue before resorting to fat stores for back up energy. As such, the more you do, the more carbs you need, and the more consistent you need to make your ingestion of them over the course of your workload.

CARBOHYDRATES (55-60%)

According to the activity levels above, these are good reference points for ranges of carbohydrate intake based on activity level:

- Low: 3–5 g/kg/day (1.36-2.27 g/lb/day)
- Medium: 5–7 g/kg/day (2.27-3.18 g/lb/day)
- High: 6–10 g/kg/day (2.72-4.55 g/lb/day)
- Extreme: 8–12 g/kg/day (3.64-5.45 g/lb/day)

(Better Health Channel 2012)

Imagine carbs like the gasoline in your car. Even better, in the case of simple carbs like sport drinks, they can act as natural and healthy *performance enhancing energy* on the spot when you are working out for long periods of time. Consult the Glycemic Index to get a better understanding of how different foods affect your blood sugar and how to use them for different needs. As much as people talk up the necessity of protein, the real foundation of any true athlete's diet is carbohydrates. Doctors, dietitians, and athletes themselves all agree.

To put this in perspective, an athletic person in good shape who weighs 68 kg (150 lbs), would need to eat between 408-680 grams per day in a high endurance or intensity workout training regimen. On the low end that translates, in easy to visualize food terms, to about 27 slices of wholegrain bread. This seems like a lot, but you wouldn't actually just eat bread! And you are doing a ton of activity, so you will need the energy.

Specializing your athletic outlet demands you also start to specialize your ingredient selection. More efficient foods will help you hit your marks with ease.

Some focal points of specializing:

- **Vegetables**– Lean into the dark green veggies! You probably don't eat enough broccoli, spinach, or some unusual choices—you could try Bok Choy!
- **Efficient vegetables**– Try adding sweet potatoes, beets, corn and such to supplement your added need for carbohydrates. Vegetables tend to be lower calorie for the value and contain fiber to help you feel fuller.
- **Grains and cereals**– Unrefined! Cook them yourself, and keep it simple—brown rice, oats, quinoa. When baking or cooking, exchange your white flour for whole grains.
- **Dairy**– Adding cottage cheese or Greek yogurt to your recipes will fill them out with excellent carbs and added protein.
- **Desserts**– Sorry, but you need to minimize sugar. Cakes, candies, and the like will slow you down. They cause massive floods of insulin that can result in terrible crashes. Especially at this stage in your training, it is recommended to lay off the goodies for your best results. (It's okay, you can cheat every now and then!)

PROTEIN (15-20%)

Don't get the wrong idea. You definitely need protein. It is *very* important for muscles and cell function. Athletes do need to eat more than the average person daily, but it does not provide the immediate and outrageous amounts of energy your body needs as you augment toward an athlete's physique. Once you reach your ideal body composition you will settle into a different ratio of nutrients. For now, you're focused on increasing volume and intensity.

To that end, gauge which tier you fall into based on:

- Average person with lower activity level: 0.8-1 g/kg/day
- Non-endurance sports: 1-1.2 g/kg/day
- High-endurance/intensity sports: 1.2-1.7 g/kg/day

(Better Health Channel 2012)

There is some research to support the timing of your protein intake. Some experts suggest that consuming protein within 15 minutes of your workout may have additional and more effective outcomes. If this works for you, it certainly doesn't hurt anything to try it. Run it against your food diary for trends, and see if it has an effect on your progress. (Murphy 2017)

A few concerns arise when considering a significant increase of protein in your diet. Obviously, if your doctor has any warnings for you based on your bloodwork, vitals, etc, take those things into consideration. For the rest of us, the only issues that commonly come up are:

- **Increased cost**– Proteins tend to be more expensive than carbs.
- **Kidneys**– Depending on what proteins you eat, and how much, there can be a potential negative impact on

kidney function. Extremely high ingestion of dietary protein can cause hypertension due to high levels of acid load on the organs, phosphate content, and some inflammation.
- **Weight**– If your choices in protein are higher in fat, they can cause undesired weight gain.
- **Exclusion**– Often, the raising of protein is confluent with insufficient intake of vegetables and other food groups. Fixation diets often lead to imbalances. (Ko, Rhee et al. 2020)

In order to broaden your base of protein options and choose the best quality of protein for your needs, try adjusting:

- **Meat**– Get only the leanest proteins possible. Chicken, some pork, and high fatty acid fish at least once a week.
- **Legumes**– These include chickpeas, black beans, lentils, kidney beans, and navy beans.
- **Soy**– Also a legume, but it is the only plant-based protein that provides a complete essential protein profile. Soy based proteins and products are a great vegetarian alternative to whey. (Despite rumors, soy protein has not been shown to lower testosterone in men. Neither does it significantly block mineral absorption, except in cases where the subject was already deficient)

FATS (25-30%)

Fat pretty much gets a bad rap because of faulty advertisement. We've already been over a lot of the reasons you need it. Remember, fat in your foods doesn't equate with getting fat. As you move to get faster and stronger you will need fat to drive that growth and help you recover.

Look for monounsaturated and polyunsaturated fats to make up the entire 30% of this macronutrient portion of your diet. These good fats can be found in:

- **Nuts**– These include almonds, pistachios, walnuts, cashews, pecans.
- **Seeds**– These include pepitas, chia seeds, flax seeds, sunflower seeds, sesame seeds.
- **Olive oil**– Use it instead of cooking oils or spreads. Mix it with vinegar for salads.
- **Avocado**– One of a kind fruit with so many good things for you.
- **Cheese**– These include feta, cottage cheese, goat cheese, gouda, ricotta, swiss, etc.
- **Dark chocolate**– We'll stress this one again. In addition to the good fat oil, it is full of antioxidants to prevent inflammation. Use it as a treat in place of sugary desserts (along with blueberries and bananas for delicious alternatives to cookies and pie!)

WATER

Water, water, water! Higher activity means higher heat which can lead to poorer bodily function. Regulate that heat and replenish your fluids constantly. A good start is roughly:

- 5-7 milliliters of water/kg/day (0.5-1 oz/lb/day)

Your urine should stay a pale yellow as a show of proper hydration.

For exercising in warmer climates, sports drinks may be

needed for proper hydration. Powdered vitamin and sodium additives can make your water more effective in higher temperatures. Retention is the key when you are pouring water out of your body in sweat.

It is very hard to gauge how much water you are losing while active, and you don't want to get into the danger zone of dehydration. Stay on top of it and continuously sip water. Pre-hydrating is also a valid technique before a competition. The main point is, do not wait until you are thirsty to drink. By that time you are already low on hydration.

Alkaline water is advertised as helping regulate the pH in your bloodstream, but there is little evidence to support a significant benefit. Most athletes just need plain old water, and lots of it.

SUPPLEMENTATION

Caffeine, although not the best thing for anyone suffering from hypertension, can be very good to help with mental acuity and to give you a zip of focus for a workout or activity. Previous worries over its diuretic nature have been put to rest in recent studies. More often than not, you are drinking caffeine in liquid, and the caffeine does not cause more excretion than you are imbibing to get it. Still, make sure you are drinking enough water with it, and avoid adding copious amounts of sugar and milk in your coffee and tea for the best results.

Besides the main source of nutrition that should be gained from food, some supplementary food products can be added for maximizing time and calorie goals. When we refer to shakes or meal replacement, we don't mean a smoothie of blended fruits and vegetables that you would have otherwise just eaten instead of drinking them. In this case, we mean powdered nutritional supplements of alternatives designed to take the place of food or give you an addition to something you struggle to consume enough of, like protein.

As you ascend toward higher levels of athleticism, it can get harder to acquire enough of the right foods because of time, energy, and money. Your diet should be your main focus, but some supplementation can serve a purpose. For the best idea of what you might add in terms of vitamins and minerals, it is recommended that you get blood work and an analysis done by a professional to address your nutritional needs. You should not blindly add significant amounts of any micronutrient for no reason. Most will not harm you, but overloading on certain vitamins can cause distress in your kidneys and liver if you don't need them.

Furthermore, excessive levels of certain vitamins can show up as a warning in a urine or blood panel for competitions and get you disqualified. Make sure you choose any additive to your diet carefully with proper research and, when possible, a doctor's approval.

THE BIG DAY

Before an event, make sure you provide your body with stable, plentiful energy with a meal one to three hours prior. This will prevent many GI issues and distress during the workload period. Use the methods you know work for you, and try them out on heavy training days to simulate the day of the event. Competition is not the time to be experimenting with new dietary trials!

Calories in your pre-event meal can range from 300-1,000 depending on time frame, duration, and intensity. For early training days, the minimum 300 calories should suffice if you wake and need to get to it. Ideally, for prolonged and intense efforts, 1,000 calories two to four hours before is even better for longevity, with a high percentage of the meal being carbohydrates. In close proximity to an event, limit fat and fiber, as they are harder to digest and will occupy oxygen and blood you need for your muscles. (American Heart Association 2015)

At a level below the drastic needs of a pro athlete, it is generally accepted that a person gets roughly one gram of carbohydrates per kilogram of body weight an hour before their workout. Pushing the meal back farther from the workout increases the intake proportionately to within three hours—two grams, two hours prior, etc. Anything past that and you will not be benefiting as much from the food you ate as it will have already been mostly digested and used.

Further, try to maintain your blood-glucose concentrations for continued output. One method of achieving this is through liquid foods, mainly carbs in the final hour before. Many athletes do better with liquids or gels in the last hour. Find out what works for your stomach and gastrointestinal stability. You can also pre-load water by drinking more over the four hours leading up to the start.

During the event, if it exceeds 90 minutes, staying hydrated and consuming 0.5 grams of carbs per pound of bodyweight every hour can help sustain proper muscle function.

After the intense physical demands, make sure you eat a full and nutrient rich meal within two hours of the event. One excellent technique for quick blood-glucose recovery is to drink equal parts freshly squeezed fruit juice and water for rapid sugar uptake. This can help avoid cramps and seizing in fatigued muscles. (Murphy 2017)

DIET AND IDEAS

There are several medical method diets, including the DASH diet for high blood pressure and hypertension, as well as the MIND diet that aims to prevent mental degradation such as dementia and Alzheimers. Both of these share some similarities with the popular

Mediterranean diet, which you may have heard of. Many of the ideas in these diets hold true to solid nutrition and good practice.

- **Vegetables**– one serving per day
- **Whole grains**– three servings per day
- **Leafy green vegetables**– six servings per week
- **Beans**– four servings per week
- **Berries**– three servings per week
- **Fish**– one plus serving per week
- **Red meat**– three servings per week max
- **Poultry**– two plus servings per week
- **Olive oil**– main cooking oil
- **Nuts**– five servings per week
- **Fried or fast food**– one serving per week max (or not at all!)
- **Alcohol, wine**– one serving per day max
- **Pastries, cake**s– four servings per week max

These are more useful guidelines to keep molding your diet into what you need to become the best. Next, we will look at how you can use this new information in your activity and raise the bar in your workouts.

CHAPTER 11
WORKING OUT

After a few years of experience, you should be doing exercises that are moderately difficult to master. Beginners tend to do lots of easy to repeat moves and there is a steep improvement with a very low learning curve at inception. And that's exactly what they need! The intermediate athlete should still mix up lots of those fundamental exercises for diversity, but you need more of a challenge.

ALL AROUND ATHLETIC

Focus on harder to learn moves and skills along with a more honed and knowledgeable routine. You will pursue less aggressive improvement in terms of making large strides, but much higher returns on specialized movements and coordination.

Moderate variability is still important, but you should be beginning to find what works more effectively for your craft. Your body knows how to respond to what you need it to do in your current shape, so you can add more difficulty.

Intermediate specs:

- Medium variability for medium training age.
- Slower gains, but higher intensity and complexity.

- Better mind-muscle connection and control. You can push yourself harder!
- Start using techniques like percentages of max output to gauge your own level and plan your workload.

("How to Train Intermediate to Advanced Athletes" 2020)

PERSPECTIVE

For example, in bicycling, beginners can just ride. Get comfortable. Mountain, road, anywhere any time. They can try to ride harder, longer. See how they feel.

Intermediate riders need to start looking at what kind of biking they want to specialize in. Researching and buying better equipment with a better understanding of the sport and their desires. Secondly, intermediate riders must add volume to their routine. Ride way more often, for longer periods of time. Be on the bike as much as possible to start really being a cyclist. (Glassford 2019)

At higher levels your routine should start to shape your life. Sleep earlier so that you can rise earlier, get that ride in before work. Prioritizing training and practice above free time and leisure.

Your riding needs to become dynamic, introducing intervals of difficulty. More acute skills like acceleration, breathing technique, cadence and rhythm need to be explored and added to your repertoire. No more sloppy form, good posture and tightening up the finer points. You get the idea. This goes for any sport you are working on. Learn the best skills from the best examples, how they do it and why you should be doing it the best way. In other words, you aren't a newbie anymore. No excuses!

DOING THE WORK

As you specialize, you will start to look at tiers of exercises a little differently. Instead of just doing overall training or compound movement, you can categorize movements in your routine into three types:

- Warm ups. No matter what level you reach, we still need to awaken our bodies with more blood flow to prevent injury.
- Preparatory exercises mimic some of the movements you will be doing, but they are more generalized and fundamental compound motions.
- The next tier involves developmental moves that directly train a competition skill (e.g. football dummy drives or footwork exercises in soccer).
- Finally, there are the master movements you will use in competition that you will train repetitiously for perfection. ("Training Beginner vs Advanced" 2021)

When it comes to intensity, think about it in percentages of max effort. If your workout is making you feel like you are only using 50%, try doing it harder, longer, heavier.

As a workout begins to feel relatively easy across the board, it's time to modify it. You can add depth, weight, or find a modified version to swap out with the standard exercise.

Instead of squats, do front squats, single leg squats, sumo squats, etc. Also think about hitting less accessed areas and which parts of the muscle you need to target for your abilities.

Start to look at strength ratios in proportion to your body size for challenges and benchmarks. The same goes for endurance and lung capacity. Athletic tests can be of great value in determining where you are. Documenting your progress, as always, is the foundation for this. Through this information you will know what you are capable of, combined with the facts of your BMI and measurements to watch progress.

Become familiar with your blood pressure and resting heart rate, plus your max effort heart rate. Comparing them to conventional average charts or getting your doctors input adds yet another layer to your expert dissection of your growth. What does homeostasis look like for you? These things will help you prevent exhaustion, injury, and illness.

If given the opportunity or if you simply choose to seek it out, have an aerobic capacity test done for oxygen uptake. This test can be extremely helpful for endurance sport athletes. Carbon dioxide and oxygen condensations show your use and efficiency of lungs and breath in this test.

Check your blood pressure and heart rate. Watch them closely and compare them to charts for averages, but also know what your natural resting state is by seeing your doctor and finding out what your homeostasis looks like for comparison. Knowing your physical tolerances and limits is very wise and applicable to your study and progress.

REP RANGES

Splits can become more complex, but don't forget your fundamentals. Sometimes a circuit of full-body exercise is still a good baseline to come back to to make sure you are still balanced and not focusing too much on an isolated muscle grouping. Incorporate a variety of reps and sets to continuously challenge yourself.

- 10-12 for midline hypertrophy with moderate weight (considered "Strength" range).
- 15-30 reps with lower weight (endurance "Burnout" range).

- Four to six reps with lots of weight (considered "Power" range).
- Lowering the weight and using bursts of explosive force at any range narrows in on fast twitch muscle activation.
- Slow, eccentric movement works into the stretch of the motion.

All of the ranges are beneficial and work your muscles. With a solid diet you will always see results from high intensity and voluminous workouts. The purpose of varying your reps is diversity of ability. Even as you begin to specialize, you have to make sure you do not have any gaps in your physique for what you need.

STAGNATING

A mistake many athletes make is only using one range of reps or style of workout for long periods of time, and they begin to see less and less visible results. This is called plateauing. Sticking with one style of workout will train your body, and you can always make it harder, but often you need a shock of unusual movement to jar your muscle memory into adapting to unknown obstacles. Use this to your advantage. You do not have to reinvent the wheel to trick your body into getting stronger. You just have to trick your body into getting stronger!

Within your sport you can find ways to drive your body to a new grade of excellence with subtle changes to your moves. Keep your desired skills in mind when you do this for the best choices.

STAYING IN STYLE

You will find which training regimens suit your needs as you gain more experience. Here are several training techniques to work into your routine to challenge your skills:

- Interval workouts are excellent for conditioning. Raising and lowering intensity and duration will prepare your body for more contingencies of workload and diversify your endurance as well as your stamina.
- Dynamic stretching– instead of static stretches, use movements to actively stretch during and after workouts. Finding new ways to reach parts of your tendons and ligaments that rarely get attention avoids repetitive fatigue and damage by loosening and activating the less occupied sections.
- Intense compound circuits– your body is a system. Every now and then, perform an intense circuit of compound motions with no breaks in between to shock your system. Think of it like a PT test for all-around athleticism. It can be eye opening for things to work on.

PRE AND POST WORKOUT FUELING

As we've gone over, eating an hour or so before a workout is optimal for professional level output. Pre-workout fasting, such as waking and immediately working out without a meal, can be dangerous if you are not used to it. Fasting in general is a very unique and risky method of dieting without the proper guidance.

Immediately following your workout, your body is primed for energy uptake, and studies show you are more nutrient receptive after high-intensity exercise. You never want to overeat, but this meal is a perfect time to eat as much as you feel you need. There is a fair amount of controversy over defeating your calories burned with an oversized meal right after working out, but in athleticism it's less about losing weight and more about energy provision.

The caloric compensation imbalances in your post-workout meal are negligible, and it was shown in an Oxford study that, in fact, no weight gains can be largely attributed to this meal in particular. Rather, the post intense workout meal is one of the most efficient and useful meals the body can obtain. The most metabolizing of useful nutrients was implemented by the subjects' bodies during this meal.

Further, the data showed that proper selection and timing of the post workout meal began to have effects on daily digestion and overall energy uptake as they maintained a consistent and abundant routine over time.

Kind of like we've mentioned before: consistency and routine make the machine run better.

Noting this, it goes to show that if you feed your workout first, and then replenish properly and generously, you will see better metabolic efficiency across your diet and a better output of energy.

In relation to nutrient metabolism, carbohydrates showed the most drastic absorption and digestion in the study. Lipids and proteins do not tend to digest much differently at any time, typically slow and steady and even more so during hard labor. The time of ingesting protein and lipids was the only factor of concern for the effect of harder digestion during the workload.

INTERMEDIATE MOVES FOR ATHLETES

Try many of these as alternates for your standard exercises for a challenge! Avoid any compromising exercises. If you feel unstable or unsure—don't do it, there are always other exercises to use, and you can always improve and try them later.

. . .

Cardio

Adding incredibly intense elements and intervals to your cardio routine will increase calorie burn and demand. This is how you work on making your metabolism more efficient. High workload, good food after.

- Burpees– Jump, hands up, squat, drop to your hands and push up, then back to squat, up, repeat!
- Battle ropes– This can act as an upper body cardio that most of us never get!
- Rowing machine (high intensity)

Legs

- Walking lunges– the most advanced form of lunges.
- Reverse sprinter lunges– eliminates compromising aspects of the forward lunge for a targeted attack on your whole leg!

Upper Body

- Twisting push ups– the horizontal adduction at the end of each side movement really gets the muscle.
- Pullovers can target the back and the chest in the last half of the motion.

Core

- There are always gaps in your core strength in some way, so try to find the weak points. All of your balance comes from your core.
- Twisting leg raises— targets obliques and offers a difficult alternative to crunches and traditional abdominal work.
- Any twisting core movement like medicine ball slams and decline Russian twists evolve your abs from single directional to multidirectionality.

Balance

Try balance-based exercises that remove your elements of control to increase your ability.

- Planks and mountain climbers— in plank, raise your knee up to your chest and clench your abs before returning the foot and repeating on the other side.
- One legged curls— your hamstrings are used to working in concert, one may be weaker than the other!
- Pistol Squats— you need to be able to stand up on one foot!
- Step ups— all around good moves for coordination and balance.

Flexibility

- Incorporate dynamic stretching.
- Yoga for unique and unusual maneuvers. You'll be surprised how difficult many can be, and how

unaccustomed you are to static holds. You can also work deeper into areas that are hard to access like your hip flexors and feet muscles.

Weak Spots

- Work on activating your shins and achilles tendons for knee stability. Toe raises and stretching the backs of your leg under the calves will help avoid ankle injury.
- Side to side lunges (skater lunges) for groin and inner knee tendon strength and full knee mobility.
- Hyperextensions and reverse hyperextensions— your lower back is your mast, but it also needs to be strong and flexible.
- Rear deltoids— the back of the shoulders are typically weaker and underdeveloped and can lead to shoulder rotator injury. Face pulls are an excellent exercise for this.
- Posture— pay close attention to your neck and how you stand and hold yourself during workouts.

PART FIVE
EXPERIENCED

CHAPTER 12
FUELING THE MACHINE

The ref is blowing the whistle. It's finally time to start the game. This is the chapter you've all been waiting for—the day of the race. (Insert another sports metaphor here.) You have muscled through all of the basics, and your knowledge is sound. Your technique is solid, and you are ready to start eating and acting like an elite athlete. The best way to do that is to break down what the professionals eat and how that applies to you and your needs. Studying the latest nutritional science and sport applications available allows us to access what their private doctors and dietitians plan for their success.

ACTING LIKE A PRO

Pro athletes have the benefit of an enforced strict diet and discipline not all of us can achieve. But, if you've reached this part of the book looking for the means to maximize your gains and athleticism, then maybe you are ready to move to the next level. The tool you will have to utilize in place of professionally supplied medical focus, is your own discipline and hard earned money to consult the experts and implement their strategies on your own.

In this section, we will exclusively explore intense athletic requirements and high level nutritional ingestion. Keep in mind, during your training periods and off-seasons you will have different and likely lower caloric needs, and much less strict rules as you make adjustments to your physique or simply maintain your athletic ability.

For a large portion of the athletic population, on a daily basis, you may not have the ability to train six hours and eat accordingly along with your day job. Pros have personal chefs, dietitians, coaches, and personal assistants who manage their schedule and routine, and they get paid to keep them on schedule. Not to mention massages, therapy, and on site clinicians to take blood and monitor micro-necessities. (Halpern 2018) Accordingly, for those who are at an advanced level in their training, this chapter will give you solid tips that can be worked into your busy life.

First, let's set the bar on what it means to be an advanced athlete in terms of calorie burn and the level of activity you're at.

LEVELING UP

As a viable comparison, MDRI (Military Dietary Reference Intakes) standards in the US military are established using averages based on athlete nutritional needs for soldiers participating in daily intense physical training. These are based around an average height and weight of 85 kg/175 cm (187 lb/ 69 in.) male and 69 kg/163 cm (152 lb/ 64 in.) female soldiers.

- 2,300 kcal/day female athletes/soldiers
- 3,250 kcal/day male athletes/soldiers

In a study published in Military Medicine, doctors compared soldiers regularly engaged in daily high volume PT to ascertain if the MDRI athlete level kcal recommendations were sufficient or excessive. The results showed a few miscalculations in terms of ratios of macronutrients being used in intense activity, but only a slightly below target calorie need as the subjects maintained bodyweight in their percentiles. (Beals, Darnell et al. 2015)

In the study, they also compared the caloric requirements for those in Special Forces, SEAL trainees, and a few other high-intensity military positions. These numbers all range higher toward 3,400 kcals/day. (Beals, Darnell et al. 2015)

All referenced training programs entail daily high volume and intensity exercises and in many cases, extreme activity equal to professional athletic competitions. Which is why most of this data is formulated around athlete performance expectations. It makes sense the two would correlate. Taking this into consideration helps to frame a basis for your caloric intake.

Let's also clarify a more concise definition of what athlete level activity entails. According to the International Sports Science Association, activity levels of a moderate athlete are considered:

- Two to three hours of intense training, five to six days a week.

High volume training generally associated with pro athletes is set at:

- Three to six hours of intense training, one to two times daily, five to six days a week.

("Nutrition and Athletic Performance" 2021)

You can easily place yourself and your training caliber according to these guidelines. This is important as you start to personalize your diet to fit the unique model you need.

PREPARATION

First and foremost, when you wake, start drinking water. You have been fasting in your sleep and need to rehydrate. This is particularly important if you plan to train soon after.

Secondly, a majority of athletes never skip breakfast. Most pro athletes eat within 30 minutes of rising in the morning. So start your day with a good meal! This may vary based on whether you intend to train right after you wake or will wait until later in the day. If you need to get right to it, limit the meal to a carb-centric 300 calories and go about your routine. If you have an hour or so, work in more protein and load as much as 1,000 calories into your breakfast.

Four qualities of the athlete diet that you need to apply to everything you eat:

- Eat high quality food.
- Eat variety—every type of nutrient.
- Eat enough. Plenty of food for plenty of work.
- Eat for your needs. Individualize your diet through careful study and tracking.

(Crowe 2021)

Let's start with discovering your needs. This comes back to that handy little food diary you should be very familiar with by now.

Your tracking does not have to be perfect and measured to the micron. But, the more you document, the more data you will have to monitor trends. Break down your diary into sections to note meaningful changes and periods.

- Time spent training
- What sport or training activity

- Calories and food eaten
- Energy levels, mood, niggles (aches and pains), and any other pertinent details (a simple one to 10 scale can be sufficient)
- Sleep quantity and quality

(Halpern 2018)

What you will be able to determine from the numbers will diagram what is and isn't working. Sluggishness may be a sign of insufficient energy, or it could be that something you added isn't sitting well with you, such as a food you have an unknown allergy to or sensitivity to.

Tracking this way, you will be able to observe ups and downs and make the meaningful differences you need to fuel competitively. You might also want to keep an eye on your meal timing to find optimal ingestion hours associated with your workouts and competitions.

Sleep tracking will show you where you are going through slumps from either not enough rest or perhaps sleeping outside the cycle of your body's ideal rhythm. You know you need sleep, regardless. If you don't sleep enough, you won't function properly. (Defining exactly how much sleep you need is, unfortunately, completely up to you and how you feel.)

Documenting every food you eat should not be a retroactive endeavor. The process needs to have forward and backward mobility to plan what you will be eating, while keeping a close watch on what you have and how it helped or hindered you.

- Plan two to three days of meals at a time.

Cook ahead to avoid deviation or laziness. If the meals are already prepped, portioned, and waiting for you, there's no tedious cooking time when you're starving, and you're less likely to grab something you shouldn't. (Measuring calories is much easier this way.)

You want to be the best, so be the best, and eat the best. Once the routine is set, it will promote itself and you staying in the zone.

PORTIONS

The average stomach is about the size of a baseball. Each meal should be about that size in volume. In order to meet caloric requirements, you may need to eat as many as six times a day without overloading in one or two meals. Remember, your post workout meal tends to be most efficient, so that meal can be a higher volume without detrimental effects.

If you need a relative scale to compare to, your diet as an advanced athlete should look a little more like:

- 50-60% Carbohydrates (up to 70% around events and during phases of raising intensity)
- 15-25% Proteins
- 20-30% Good fats

As always, we'll reiterate that personalization completely allows for variation on these ratios. Your doctor and dietitian, your physiology and biology may all have some things to tell you about how to adjust if you get checked out.

BODY COMPOSITION

Body fat percentages and acceptable ranges differ greatly for individual sports. Some elements of healthy body ratios also have to do with your body type, blood levels, and genetics. Seek out guidance from your doctor for extremely precise management of body fat and musculature. Failure to do so can result in dangerous deficiencies.

Increasing lean body mass can be observed over four to 12 weeks of consistent protein increase and regimented progressive overload resistance training. Long term, steady gains are the most durable and sustainable.

There are some unfortunate facts you have to be aware of:

- You cannot grow muscle fiber and lose fat at the same time.
- You can and should try to maintain muscle mass while losing fat—which is ideal.

You can also grow lean muscle without gaining much fat, but gains are gains and losses are losses. You're either in a deficit of calories and losing weight, or you are in an abundance of calories and growing.

REQUIREMENTS FOR SPORTS

Average individuals who engage in light to moderate activity typically require 25-35 calories/kg/day (11.3-16 kcal /lb/day). Advanced athletes can require as much as 40-70 calories/kg/day.

The International Society of Sports Nutrition prescribes relative caloric needs for:

- 50-100 kg athletes: 2,000-7,000 kcal/day
- 100-150 kg athletes: 6,000-12,000 kcal/day

(Economos et al. 1993)

These estimates are broad based on the supposed demands of professional level competition and training. The differences in body types, BMI, and other factors demand a range of caloric needs in the figures.

Endurance runners, for example, exhibit lower costs of energy for efficient movement from lighter bodies which displace their mass over a larger area through perpetual motion.

Acceleration, especially from a stop, is more prevalent in explosive strength athletes, as well as in sprinters. These conditions change the required energy and the rate of use for different athletes.

MEAL TIMING

A general guideline for most athletes to follow:

- Strength athletes should eat protein and possibly carbohydrates around four hours before exercise and no more than two hours after. This tends to optimize nitrogen conditions and protein synthesis in the muscles.
- In the case of endurance athletes, smaller amounts of protein are recommended with mostly carbohydrates between one to four hours prior.
- Balance and flexibility heavy athletes should base their intake around those parameters based on the execution of their typical movements. If they require longevity, use the endurance parameters. For optimal force, use strength.

More than anything, the timing for your best results is what more and more dietitians are stressing. You do not want to run out of juice in the middle of a work out.

HYDRATION

We cannot stress enough the need to properly and sufficiently hydrate. Athletes should strive to maintain *euhydration*, meaning thorough hydration, before, during, and after an event to avoid heat illness or other issues. Train yourself to hydrate by:

- Continuously sipping
- Drink when you are not thirsty

That being said, there are a few scenarios when hyper-hydrating or purposeful dehydration can be very detrimental to your performance. Some athletes over hydrate, causing necessary, excessive urination. Lowered sodium levels will also lead to a lowered capacity for water retention.

Dehydrating to meet weight for an event can have negative effects on your performance. This will indelibly behave in a similar fashion to your meal timing, as you begin to understand how close to competition you need to cease or slow water consumption. Officially, using glycerol and some other additives to retain water has been banned in professional sports as doping. *For euhydration, drink roughly five to 10 ml/kg (two to four ml/lb) during the four hours leading up to an event.

E = ENERGY

We've discussed glycogen in muscles, and what that really does is activate muscle contraction. It is an energy *substrate* (chemical activator) with that exact purpose, so as we act, we deplete it slowly over time. Even though you digest less when under stress, eating simple carbs can counter this depletion.

Ultimately, to increase endurance via nutrition, you must increase or maintain glycogen stores in muscles. Over time, dietary training can see skeletal muscle and the liver growing a slightly deeper reserve.

For a more immediate saturation and a sort of muscle conditioning phase, this method can help raise and maintain glycogen levels temporarily without many adverse effects.

- Six days out from competition, eat a low carb diet for three days.
- Three days from the event, switch to a high carb diet.
- Combine with more citrate in your diet, which decreases glycolysis (the acidic metabolic breakdown of sugars) It can be found in lemons, limes, grapefruit, and oranges.

This can increase your stores by about one and a half times.

This technique should not be implemented constantly, but can be implemented for special case performance. Further, glycogen optimization only works for longevity. Think of it like getting a temporarily bigger gas tank. The car runs longer on a bigger tank, but more duration doesn't mean more power. Fuel is fuel, not boost. Loading in this fashion serves less purpose for strength athletes. *Make sure you test this method of loading well before the week of the event on lower stakes training days.

Tip– Right before and during a prolonged workout, only take simple monosaccharides or oligosaccharides. They will kick in a short while into the event and this will sustain performance. These can be found optimally in fruits, sports drinks, and carb gels.

Throughout a prolonged workload of three to four hours, maintaining liver glycogen stores is optimal to avoid fatigue and crashing.

For best results, use a six to eight percent glucose solution in liquid periodically. Too much sugar and you can trick your system into occupying resources for digestion instead of athletic needs. This can also cause dehydration.

CARRYING YOUR CARBOHYDRATES

Carbohydrates carry an energy value of about four kcals per gram of food (~4 Kcal/g). (UW Health 2019)

Advanced athlete carbohydrate demands:

- Eight to 10 grams of carbs/kg/day (3.6-4.5 grams/lb/day)

(Clifford, Maloney 2008)

Combinations– The main source of fuel for muscles is glycogen, provided most noticeably by consumed carbohydrates. This should comprise at least 55-60% of your diet near competition, if not a bit more. To offset this high intake of carbs, if you are training toward a lower energy diet plan, lower your fat intake to below 25%. Conversely, if you are on a high energy diet, pair the high carbs with high fats around 30%.

Terms of use– The first thing to get used up are the carbs/sugar in the bloodstream, then the backup stores in muscle glycogen, then fat. So, you need to get those levels back up after an event, (or during longer activities).

For a quick post event snack try:

- Half cup of granola
- One to two ounces of baked snack like pretzels

- Eight to 16 ounces of a sport drink

Tip– While fructose in a standard diet can lead to issues in high concentrations of simple sugar, in the case of endurance running and the like, fructose has been shown to generate less of an insulin response than other forms of sugar. Insulin inhibits lipid metabolism and increases glycolysis, so minimizing it can promote retention of glycogen stores in muscles, instead of promoting lactic acid build up which inhibits muscle contraction. Try mixing these into your water (in moderation):

- Apple juice
- Agave syrup
- Honey
- Molasses

Over 90 minutes– During higher demand and intensity competitions, drink liquid carbs and electrolytes to replenish glycogen for consistency. This applies to sustained effort and for repeated sprints and taxing bursts. For best results, ingest routinely, around every 15-20 minutes if the event will last longer than 90 minutes.

Response training– In training practices some results have been shown for cellular adaptation. Many athletes *train low*, in a slight deficit of carbohydrates, to alter glycogen tendencies in the muscle. This is what is referred to as adaptive response. Similar to the event loading, adaptive response training aims to maximize the muscle's capability to retain and store glycogen. Not everyone will react positively to it. Make small adjustments and track your reactions carefully!

Fiber carbs– Fiber needs to be carefully monitored for consistency. You do need it, but upping or lowering it can have drastic effects on both your GI and your performance. Always slowly increase your fiber intake progressively and give your body time to adjust before augmenting.

Use your food diary to keep track of your excretions to help you find your ideal regularity.

PROTEIN LIKE A PRO

Protein offers roughly the same value as carbohydrates with around four calories per gram (~4 Kcal/g). (UW Health 2019)

Protein is very necessary for growth, but elevated protein diets primarily benefit strength training, otherwise it can be an excess in your diet. For most growth phases, you simply need to increase calories in any form (best quality foods, of course).

- 1.2-2 grams of protein/kg/day (0.5-1 gram/lb/day)

(Clifford, Maloney 2008)

While higher intakes of protein seem to be most necessary in short spans when intensifying training or reducing energy intake, the consensus is that athletes need more than the average person. About double, actually.

Bodybuilders and extreme weight workload athletes may need significantly more protein. By creating a nitrogen positive balance through raised protein intake, the overall nitrogen content in the blood pool will promote substrate growth and increase the demand for and production of muscle fiber.

Caution– Excess protein is excreted predominantly in urine. As such, too much can cause kidney and bladder stress. As always, slow increases will prevent strained digestion if you are not accustomed to consuming so many protein packed foods.

But are you getting enough? Tracking your weight, strength, and BMI can help determine if you are getting enough protein. *Catabolism* can cause muscle wasting over time if you are receiving insufficient nutrients. If you begin to lose muscle mass, you need to up your intake to accommodate your level of effort. Additional calories may be a solution, regardless of nutrient type.

Bouncing back– Eating protein soon after an event or training session has shown signs of better recovery of athletic muscle function and reduced onset muscle soreness. Insulin, which is released during digestion, promotes protein synthesis. While the hormone can cause performance hindrances before or during an event, insulin is very helpful afterwards.

Moreover, many athletes experience similar results from ingesting 20-30g of protein during exercise. Although, eating while trying to workout is not always ideal. Either way, an improved balance of nitrogen will increase muscular and total body protein synthesis.

Whey– One method of increasing blood level amino acids is to eat or drink easily digested whey protein supplements to add to your growth. This source of protein is also naturally high in glutamine and BCAAs. *Be certain to research what is in your powdered supplements. Production lines are not always clean or pure, and many companies add extensive micronutrients and chemicals that you may not want or need.

FUNCTIONS OF FAT

Fat molecules are much denser macronutrients and provide around nine kcals per gram (~9 Kcal/g). (UW Health 2019)

- 1.2-1.4 grams of fat/kg/day (~0.6 gram/lb/day) (Endurance)
- 1.6-1.7 grams of fat/kg/day (~0.75 gram/lb/day) (Strength)

(Clifford, Maloney 2008)

Fats can be used as fuel, but this usually depends on your biochemistry and how long you typically exercise for. There is a breaking point once you deplete certain available resources in your body, and your system will turn on fat stores and fat foods to function. Training your body to do this needs to be done cautiously so as not to over exhaust yourself.

Although we have stated not to over do it on fats the day of an event, fats are essential to proper brain function and hormone production. You won't sleep well or develop properly without them. Consuming fats with protein and carbohydrates post-event is optimal.

If you need to drop weight, lowering calorie-dense, fatty foods will help, just be sure you do not drop too far below the 20% mark. Your neural systems depend on fat.

SUPPLEMENTS

We all would love to pop a pill and get the best results, and there is a lot of false advertising out there about professional supplements that claim to do just that. More often than not, these products do very little, if not some harm—like putting stress on your processing systems. Real athletes primarily just eat food!

If you decide to add something to your diet, whether based on your own research or your doctor's, keep a close eye on your food diary for performance indicators to see if there is any negative or positive effect from the new addition.

STIMULATING SUBSTANCES

Both creatine and caffeine have been shown to possess benefits if used in moderation. Caffeine is almost always found in beverages rich in antioxidants and has displayed beneficial attributes contributing to mental acuity and increased focus in exercise concentration.

Creatine is a natural chemical produced in the body that we use to make ATP in anaerobic conditions in our cells. We also ingest creatine from fish and red meats. Skeletal muscles with raised creatine have shown more protein synthesis activity, glycogen retention, and strength endurance. However, creatine can be tough on your kidneys and liver, like any excess of unused proteins, so ingest creatine supplements with caution.

Be wary of many supplements like these. While there is some evidence to support their efficacy, the results are somewhat negligible. Many doctors and dietitians dismiss them completely.

- **Glutamine**– A naturally abundant building block for making proteins in the body.

- **BCAAs** (Branch-Chain Amino Acids)– Stimulate protein synthesis in muscles.
- **Arginine**– Another protein building amino acid.
- **Phosphatidic acid**– Responsible for cell signaling and communication in the body.
- **Adenosine-triphosphate**– Chemical bond that drives processes in cells.

All of these chemicals occur naturally within us or in foods, and are necessary to perform bodily function. However, adding them in refined forms has very debatable results. The safest way to acquire all of your nutrients is through food.

Lastly, it might go without saying that alcohol is not the best thing for your body. It is essentially poison in large quantities, even if it also acts as a stimulant. Also, it is very calorie dense. Alcohol marks about seven kcals per gram. (UW Health 2019)

CONDITIONAL CALORIES

Other factors may contribute to your caloric and hydration requirements during performance. Especially when traveling for an event, carefully research and train for the local environmental effects on your event.

Altitude– Your competition might be at a higher altitude than you are used to. This will affect your oxygen uptake drastically. You will also burn far more calories as your body works harder to perform functions.

Extreme cold or heat– Apparel is the first line of defense for both the cold to prevent freezing and blocking the harsh rays of the sun that can cause you to burn and overheat. Both scenarios are similar in that they will demand much higher quantities of water and food to maintain all of your athletic functions.

Vegetarianism/Special diets– Vegetarian and vegan athletes should unquestionably work with a dietitian for the safest and best results. Vegetarian diets have shown risks of low protein, creatine, carnosine, fatty acids, low iron and riboflavin. Restrictive diets in general must be carefully navigated to avoid deficiencies and damages to vital systems.

Ergogenic aids– If you eat the right diet, you should not need an excess of additives. As an athlete, your body works better than the average system, and is much more efficient to begin with.

Supplemental nutrition– For ease of access and use, many products are designed in gels and race day packets. Examine the ingredients for best results.

RECOVERY

No matter how elite you become, you will always need a day off every now and then to recover. Not only for your body, but for your mind. We need diversion and comfort to maintain healthy perspectives. For lack of a better word, these can also be cheat days where you indulge in some foods that you normally would not during your strict training. Around competition it is recommended to refrain from this behavior.

Treat yourself. If you choose to veer from your diet one day a week, an excess of calories won't mess you up cumulatively.

Realize though, that you are not accustomed to eating junk food and you may feel sluggish the following day if you overdo it.

Even if you do not deviate from your diet, you should still enjoy holistic regrouping of some sort. A break from your routine will not ruin you. At least one day a week, consider taking a day off to alleviate stress from your brain. This can be an active recovery day through yoga or tai chi, or another diversion. For some, it simply means sitting on the couch and reading a good book!

CHAPTER 13
TRAINING

As a professional athlete, we won't tell you exactly what to do, you have a trainer or you know your sport better than anybody by now. However, there are advanced techniques that can match your expertise with equivalent level moves. For those of you who are just coming into their own as athletes, along with the self taught, there is never too much information to add options to your workout program.

Athlete training exercises should fall into these four brackets:

- **Fundamental**– Moves that use your whole system and keep you optimally functional.
- **Training to train**– Strength, endurance, flexibility, balance. Specialized growth exercises.
- **Training to compete**– Moves that augment and hone your in-competition skills.
- **Training to win**– Only the specific moves you will use in an event.

Thinking of your workouts this way will help you decide what is essential or not necessary. The more specialized you become, the more specific your routine and training will get.

A gymnast does not really need to strengthen his throwing arm. Not to say cross training is not useful. Adjacent skill building can be very helpful to round out a skill set, but by and large, if you get too far afield from your study, you are only stunting your progress.

As you become more refined, you will notice some diminishing returns. This is natural. Forging a knife requires altering the shape of the metal, but sharpening the knife once it is made is almost imperceptible to the naked eye. But the blade can always get sharper!

Do not despair if you gain less the better you get. It will demand more time and energy, and more dynamic, detailed attention to the methods you use to perfect your physique.

The positive trade off is that you won't need to make massive strides any longer once you are at peak performance for your sport. You must focus on honing your skill as opposed to raw gains. Plateaus still exist at your level, but you shouldn't need to make huge changes if you have found your optimal body composition for your sport.

ADVANCED OUTLOOK

To use cycling as an example again, this is what an advanced rider's program might look like compared with the intermediate cyclist reference in the previous section.

Riding at or around 75% of your max heart rate while being able to talk with other riders is a good sign you need to up your intensity. (Glassford 2019)

Intense interval training is the most common method of keeping your workouts from being too long and hard for wear and tear, and getting the extreme workload you need.

This goes for many other sports and athletics. Try shorter

bursts of intensity with intermittent breaks of moderate sustained effort, without dropping into low level activity.

ADAPTATION

Strength adaptation deals largely with the mind and the neural functions accommodating your physical demands and firing appropriately. Workload alters your muscle fiber composition over time, increasing or solidifying your strength capacity. Muscle contraction, intensity, and duration should be the focus of your strength training to make significant progress and beat out stagnation. (Tobin 2014)

Power/acceleration tends to be based on reflected inhibition and facilitation. A lot of this training needs to focus on antagonistic muscle activation in concert with your major muscle response. In other words, contrasting forces coordinate for maximum output. This means a better connection between multi joint moves and variable repetition. Using lighter loads will help teach your neural response to fire more explosive muscle command and promote bursting motion and ability. (Tobin 2014)

THREE METHODS OF BREAKING A STALL

Use of these techniques are ideally implemented by advanced athletes with a baseline of five years of resistance training. Optimally, this experience would also incorporate elevated strength levels in proportional power, such as squatting twice one's bodyweight. These advanced methods can also be used with supervision by anyone who is no longer benefiting from a traditional training regimen and experiencing a plateau in their gains.

VRT (Variable Resistance Training)

Three types of curves exist in resistance exercises:

- **Ascending curve**– Lifting more in the latter half of the motion (bench press, squat).
- **Descending curve**– More weight is lifted in the first part of the move (upright row, chin up).
- **Bell shaped curve**– More common in isolation, single-joint moves. The most weight is possible in the middle of the move (bicep curl, hamstring curl).

Involve resistance bands or chains to supplant the traditional curve in the motion. Resistance will make the entire action difficult, optimizing muscle twitch.

Eccentric Training

This is also called negative training as it focuses on the back end of an exercise. It is also often the most neglected part of a move. We can actually perform 20-60% more in eccentric parts of exercises than the concentric. Imagine lowering yourself from a pull up. You may not be able to pull yourself back up to the top, but you can always let yourself down slowly. Many eccentric focused moves require assistance, a partner, or resistance bands.

Over-Speed

Over-speeding also involves assisted movements, but to relieve weight and co-activation. Though it seems counterintuitive, allowing muscles to do things you normally could not do by assisting them actually trains muscles to learn how to accomplish a move you struggle with.

For example, jump training with a harness or bands has shown evidence of extensive gains in vertical jump height. Studies have shown an estimated average of 10% increase in ability from this concentrated training.

("How to Train Intermediate to Advanced Athletes" 2020)

A few other methods you might try to challenge your athletic prowess and something new:

- **Super-sets**– Back to back pairings of exercises with no rest between.
- **Drop-sets**– Continuous sets with ever-dropping weight until the least weight is near impossible due to muscle failure.
- **High rep/low rep**– A burn-out, muscle-shocking method of using less reps and higher weight for the first few sets, followed by a final set of lower weight with a high volume of reps.
- **HIIT** (High Intensity Interval Training)– Executes sets at maximum output, with only a timed break in between to recover.

You finally have all the training tips and tools you need, and more importantly you have all the food you need to do it right.

FINAL WORDS

There is no ready-in-minutes microwave solution to making the incredible vehicle that is your body work better, but it is worth it to take the time and find the right food. It's an exciting, delicious, and worthy challenge. Your success depends on it.

Perfecting your diet will perfect your body. The best machine demands the best fuel. The vast sum of information you now have available will provide you with the means to make the instrumental changes in your dietary life that will propel you to athletic greatness.

Nutrition has come a long way in a short span of time, and so have you. You have the benefit of living during the outstanding results of the renaissance of sports nutrition. Medical science is extremely advanced and thorough, and studies into the health of the brain and the connection between the mind and body are growing exponentially. The human body is no longer a mysterious machine. It's still an amazing one, though. And you have access to unlimited knowledge and many free learning tools.

Let this book act as a guidepost for the ultimate strategy on fine tuning your fuel. Use your Food and Performance Diary. It will be your best friend, coach, and support group all in one! Note every detail, ask yourself the hard questions, and be honest. How were you feeling during this workout? What exercise was harder, easier, where was your head at? What state was your body in? Did you notice a specific change you made that helped or hindered you?

Pay attention to what your body is trying to tell you. It may seem like a lot, but you perform impressive feats on the field and on the track all the time. Now you will do more, at a higher level than you ever thought possible.

This is the way for an aspiring athlete to behave like a pro athlete—and to become a pro athlete. We'll meet you in the kitchen after the race!

Ask yourself this one thing as you cross the finish line:

"What should I have for lunch?"

Subscribe now at the link below to receive a bonus guide with:

- Nutritional fun facts
- Sports statistics and records
- Funny crossovers between them all

https://www.books.house/sports-health-guide-opt-in

If you enjoyed this book, please review it on Amazon. Thank you!

REFERENCES

American Heart Association. 2015. "Food as Fuel Before, during and after Workouts." Www.heart.org. 2015. https://www.heart.org/en/healthy-living/healthy-eating/eat-smart/nutrition-basics/food-as-fuel-before-during-and-after-workouts.

Andati, Bryan. 2018. Review of *Sports Nutrition; a Historical Perspective*. Web.colby.edu. GLOBAL FOOD, HEALTH, AND SOCIETY. October 28, 2018. https://web.colby.edu/st297-global18/2018/10/28/sports-nutrition-a-historical-perspective/.

Aoi, Wataru, Yuji Naito, and Toshikazu Yoshikawa. 2006. "Exercise and Functional Foods." *Nutrition Journal* 5 (1). https://doi.org/10.1186/1475-2891-5-15.

"Athletic Body Type: Getting into the Nitty Gritty of Attaining This Body Shape." 2021. BetterMe Blog. January 21, 2021. https://betterme.world/articles/athletic-body-type/.

Ayuda, Tiffany. 2018. "The Top 11 Nutrients Your Body Needs to Build Muscle." Life by Daily Burn. February 28, 2018. https://dailyburn.com/life/health/top-nutrients-build-muscle/.

"Balance." 2022. Wikipedia. February 22, 2022. https://en.wikipedia.org/wiki/Balance_.

Beals, Kim, Matthew E. Darnell, Mita Lovalekar, Rachel A. Baker, Takashi Nagai, Thida San-Adams, and Michael D. Wirt.

2015. "Suboptimal Nutritional Characteristics in Male and Female Soldiers Compared to Sports Nutrition Guidelines." *Military Medicine* 180 (12): 1239–46. https://doi.org/10.7205/MILMED-D-14-00515.

"Better Health Channel. 2012. "Sporting Performance and Food." Vic.gov.au. 2012. https://www.betterhealth.vic.gov.au/health/healthyliving/sporting-performance-and-food.

Bjarnadottir, Adda MS. 2017. "25 Simple Tips to Make Your Diet Healthier." Healthline. Healthline Media. November 6, 2017. https://www.healthline.com/nutrition/healthy-eating-tips.

Brown, Laura. 2022. "Changing Your Diet Could Add Ten Years to Your Life – New Research." The Conversation. February 8, 2022. https://theconversation.com/changing-your-diet-could-add-ten-years-to-your-life-new-research-176494.

"Calories Burned during Fitness." 2017. OnHealth. July 13, 2017. https://www.onhealth.com/content/1/calories_burned_during_fitness.

CDC. 2019. "Body Mass Index (BMI)." Centers for Disease Control and Prevention. 2019. https://www.cdc.gov/healthyweight/assessing/bmi/index.html.

"Change Diet, Exercise Habits at Same Time for Best Results, Study Says." News Center. 2013. https://med.stanford.edu/news/all-news/2013/04/change-diet-exercise-habits-at-same-time-for-best-results-study-says.html.

Cleveland Clinic. 2016. "Eating & Psychology | Cleveland Clinic." Cleveland Clinic. 2016. https://my.clevelandclinic.org/health/articles/10681-the-psychology-of-eating.

Clifford, J, and K Maloney. 2008. "Nutrition for the Athlete - 9.362 - Extension." Extension. 2008. https://extension.colostate.edu/topic-areas/nutrition-food-safety-health/nutrition-for-the-athlete-9-362/.

Colby College. 2013. Review of *Anatomy of the Athlete*.

Https://Www.colby.edu. Colby College. January 7, 2013. https://www.colby.edu/chemistry/BC176/Anatomy.pdf.

"Compound vs. Isolation Exercises: Benefits and Differences." 2018. 8fit. Accessed April 5, 2022. https://8fit.com/fitness/compound-vs-isolation-exercises-benefits-and-differences.

Crowe, Tim. 2021. "What pro Athletes Really Eat | Live Better." Medibank Live Better. April 15, 2021. https://www.medibank.com.au/livebetter/be-magazine/exercise/what-elite-athletes-really-eat/.

"Definition of MUSCULATURE." 2022. Www.merriam-Webster.com. Accessed April 5, 2022. https://www.merriam-webster.com/dictionary/musculature.

"Definition of PHYSIQUE." 2022. Www.merriam-Webster.com. Accessed April 5, 2022. https://www.merriam-webster.com/dictionary/physique.

Economos, Christina D., Sharon S. Bortz, and Miriam E. Nelson. 1993. "Nutritional Practices of Elite Athletes." *Sports Medicine* 16 (6): 381–99. https://doi.org/10.2165/00007256-199316060-00004.

"Eight Essential Nutrients for Bone and Joint Health - Craig Castleman Greene, MD, MBA." 2022. Www.craigcgreenemd.com. https://www.craigcgreenemd.com/blog/eight-essential-nutrients-for-bone-and-joint-health.

"Endurance." 2020. Wikipedia. April 21, 2020. https://en.wikipedia.org/wiki/Endurance.

"Exercise and Eating Healthy." 2014. Healthline. 2014. https://www.healthline.com/health/fitness-exercise-eating-healthy.

"Fat Facts, the Right Amount for a Healthy Diet." 2021. Penn State Extension. July 19, 2021. https://extension.psu.edu/fat-facts-the-right-amount-for-a-healthy-diet.

Fitzgerald, Dylan. 2004. "Nutrition for Weight Loss: What You Need to Know about Fad Diets." Familydoctor.org. February 19, 2004. https://familydoctor.org/nutrition-weight-loss-need-know-fad-diets/#.

"Flexibility | Sports Medicine | UC Davis Health." Ucdavis.edu. 2014. https://health.ucdavis.edu/sportsmedicine/resources/flexibility_descriprion.html.

"Four Pillars of Mental Fitness." 2019. US. May 29, 2019. https://wellbeing.lifeworks.com/blog/four-pillars-of-mental-fitness/.

Franziska Spritzler, RD, CDE. 2018. "10 Magnesium-Rich Foods That Are Super Healthy." Healthline. Healthline Media. August 22, 2018. https://www.healthline.com/nutrition/10-foods-high-in-magnesium.

Glassford, Peter. 2019. "Beginner, Intermediate or Advanced? What Training Should You Focus On?" Consummate Athlete. November 30, 2019. https://consummateathlete.com/beginner-intermediate-or-advanced-what-training-should-you-focus-on/.

Gunnars, Kris. 2017. "10 High-Fat Foods That Are Actually Super Healthy." Healthline. 2017. https://www.healthline.com/nutrition/10-super-healthy-high-fat-foods.

Gunnars, Kris. 2018. "22 High-Fiber Foods You Should Eat." Healthline. 2018. https://www.healthline.com/nutrition/22-high-fiber-foods.

Halpern, Marc. 2018. "What Elite Athletes Eat (and Do) That You Should Too (or Not)." Whole Life Challenge. January 15, 2018. https://www.wholelifechallenge.com/what-elite-athletes-eat-and-do-you-should-too-or-not/.

Harvard Health Publishing. 2016. "Micronutrients Have Major Impact on Health - Harvard Health." Harvard Health. Harvard Health. September 6, 2016. https://www.health.harvard.edu/staying-healthy/micronutrients-have-major-impact-on-health.

Harvard School of Public Health. 2012. "Vitamin E." The Nutrition Source. September 18, 2012. https://www.hsph.harvard.edu/nutritionsource/vitamin-e/.

Harvard. 2012. "Vitamin C." The Nutrition Source. September

18, 2012. https://www.hsph.harvard.edu/nutritionsource/vitamin-c/.

"Healthy Eating Plan." 2019. Nih.gov. 2019. https://www.nhlbi.nih.gov/health/educational/lose_wt/eat/calories.htm.

"How to Determine the Best Macronutrient Ratio for Your Goals." 2016. Www.acefitness.org. April 15 2016. Accessed April 6, 2022. https://www.acefitness.org/resources/pros/expert-articles/5904/how-to-determine-the-best-macronutrient-ratio-for-your-goals/.

"How to Maintain and Improve Physical Balance." 2018. Https://Taylorpilatesandfitness.com. https://taylorpilatesandfitness.com/blog/how-to-maintain-and-improve-physical-balance/.

"How to Train Intermediate to Advanced Athletes." 2020. SimpliFaster. September 23, 2020. https://simplifaster.com/articles/training-intermediate-advanced-athletes/.

"How to Use Common Isolation Exercises." 2021. Verywell Fit. April 29, 2021. https://www.verywellfit.com/isolation-exercises-description-3498374.

Institute of Medicine (US) Subcommittee on Interpretation and Uses of Dietary Reference Intakes, and Institute of Medicine (US) Standing Committee on the Scientific Evaluation of Dietary Reference Intakes. 2012. "Introduction to Dietary Planning." Nih.gov. National Academies Press (US). 2012. https://www.ncbi.nlm.nih.gov/books/NBK221366/.

Jeffrey C. Ives, Kristin Neese, Nick Downs, Harrison Root, Tim Finnerty. 2020. "The Effects of Competitive Orientation on Performance in Competition." The Sport Journal. February 21, 2020. https://thesportjournal.org/article/the-effects-of-competitive-orientation-on-performance-in-competition/.

Jennings, Kerri-Ann. 2017. "11 Best Foods to Boost Your Brain and Memory." Healthline. May 9, 2017. https://www.healthline.com/nutrition/11-brain-foods.

Ko, Gang-Jee, Connie M. Rhee, Kamyar Kalantar-Zadeh, and Shivam Joshi. 2020. "The Effects of High-Protein Diets on Kidney Health and Longevity." *Journal of the American Society of Nephrology* 31 (8): ASN.2020010028. https://doi.org/10.1681/asn.2020010028.

Leal, Darla. 2015. "Is Nutrition More Important than Exercise?" Verywell Fit. Verywell Fit. July 24, 2015. https://www.verywellfit.com/nutrition-vs-exercise-80-nutrition-wins-3121406.

Leal, Darla. 2018. "An Overview of Sports Nutrition." Verywell Fit. Verywellfit. February 5, 2018. https://www.verywellfit.com/fitness-sports-nutrition-4157142.

"List of Gymnastic Events." n.d. SportsRec. https://www.sportsrec.com/7829612/list-of-gymnastic-events.

Medline Plus. 2015. "Nutrition and Athletic Performance: MedlinePlus Medical Encyclopedia." Medlineplus.gov. 2015. https://medlineplus.gov/ency/article/002458.htm.

MedlinePlus. 2019. "Carbohydrates." Medlineplus.gov. National Library of Medicine. 2019. https://medlineplus.gov/carbohydrates.html.

"Mental Fitness Explained by a CBT Psychologist." 2019. Starling Minds. October 27, 2019. https://www.starlingminds.com/mental-fitness-explained-by-a-cbt-psychologist/.

"Michael Phelps' 10000 Calories Diet: What the American Swimmer Ate While Training for Beijing Olympics?" 2021. Olympics.com. May 16, 2021. https://olympics.com/en/featured-news/michael-phelps-10000-calories-diet-what-the-american-swimmer-ate-while-training-.

Milner, Clare E. 2008. *Functional Anatomy for Sport and Exercise : Quick Reference*. London ; New York: Routledge.

Mozaffarian, Dariush, Irwin Rosenberg, and Ricardo Uauy. 2018. "History of Modern Nutrition Science—Implications for Current Research, Dietary Guidelines, and Food Policy." *BMJ* 361 (June): k2392. https://doi.org/10.1136/bmj.k2392.

Murphy, Lee. 2017. "Nutrient Timing: Pre and Post-Workout

Questions Answered!" Blog.nasm.org. https://blog.nasm.org/workout-and-nutrition-timing.

"Muscle | Systems, Types, Tissue, & Facts." 2019. In *Encyclopædia Britannica*. https://www.britannica.com/science/muscle.

Newman, Tim. 2020. "Nutrition: Nutrients and the Role of the Dietitian and Nutritionist." Www.medicalnewsday.com. January 9, 2020. https://www.medicalnewsday.com/articles/160774.

Newman, Tim. 2020. "Nutrition: Nutrients and the Role of the Dietitian and Nutritionist." Www.medicalnewsday.com. January 9, 2020. https://www.medicalnewsday.com/articles/160774.

"Nutrition and Athletic Performance: What to Consider." 2021. Www.medicalnewsday.com. April 20, 2021. https://www.medicalnewsday.com/articles/nutrition-for-athletes#importance.

"Nutrition and Physical Activity." 2020. Myhealth.alberta.ca. September 10, 2020. https://myhealth.alberta.ca/health/pages/conditions.aspx?Hwid=ta1294.

"Nutrition for Tendon and Ligament Health." 2016. Rejoov-Wellness. February 19, 2016. https://rejoovwellness.com/nutrition-for-tendon-and-ligament-health/.

"Nutritional Science." 2021. Wikipedia. September 7, 2021. https://en.wikipedia.org/wiki/Nutritional_science.

"Origins and History of Sport Nutrition." n.d. Human Kinetics. https://us.humankinetics.com/blogs/excerpt/origins-and-history-of-sport-nutrition.

"Physical Strength." 2020. Wikipedia. March 20, 2020. https://en.wikipedia.org/wiki/Physical_strength.

"Physical Strength: Why It's Important & How to Increase It!" 2020. Lean Squad. February 5, 2020. https://lean-squad.com/blog/physical-strength-why-its-important-how-to-increase-it/.

Psychology, Nutritional. 2022. "Diet and Mental Health - the Center for Nutritional Psychology." Nutritional Psychology.

February 26, 2022. https://www.nutritional-psychology.org/what-is-nutritional-psychology/.

"Push-Pull Workouts: Routines and Guide for Building Muscle." 2020. Healthline. September 29, 2020. https://www.healthline.com/nutrition/push-pull-workout.

Raman, Ryan. 2019. "The 8 Best Diet Plans — Sustainability, Weight Loss, and More." Healthline. Healthline Media. August 5, 2019. https://www.healthline.com/nutrition/best-diet-plans.

Ron, M. 1995. "Nutrition and Exercise--a Consensus View." *Asia Pacific Journal of Clinical Nutrition* 4 Suppl 1 (November): 34–38. https://pubmed.ncbi.nlm.nih.gov/24398242/.

"Small Changes in Diet Could Help You Live Healthier, More Sustainably." 2021. University of Michigan News. August 18, 2021. https://news.umich.edu/small-changes-in-diet-could-help-you-live-healthier-more-sustainably/.

"Small Changes in Diet Could Help You Live Healthier, More Sustainably." 2021. University of Michigan News. August 18, 2021. https://news.umich.edu/small-changes-in-diet-could-help-you-live-healthier-more-sustainably/.

"Sport and Competition | Psychology Today." 2019. Psychology Today. 2019. https://www.psychologytoday.com/us/basics/sport-and-competition.

"Sports Nutrition, Definition, Purpose, History, Description." n.d. Reference.jrank.org. Accessed April 5, 2022. https://reference.jrank.org/fitness/Sports_Nutrition.html.

"Stiffness." 2022. Wikipedia. March 26, 2022. https://en.wikipedia.org/wiki/Flexibility_.

"The Importance of Good Physical Balance." 2016. Azumio.com. 2016. https://www.azumio.com/blog/fitness/importance-of-physical-balance.

"The Push/Pull/Legs Routine for Muscle Gains | Aston University." 2016. Www.aston.ac.uk. https://www.aston.ac.uk/sport/news/tips/fitness-exercise/push-pull-legs.

REFERENCES 167

Tobin, Daniel P. 2014. "Advanced Strength and Power Training for the Elite Athlete." *Strength and Conditioning Journal* 36 (2): 59–65. https://doi.org/10.1519/ssc.0000000000000044.

Training Beginner vs Advanced Sprint Athletes | Sprinting-Workouts.com." 2021. Sprinting Workouts | Training for Speed & Power. February 14, 2021. Accessed April 7, 2022. https://sprintingworkouts.com/blogs/training/beginner-advanced-athlete-training.

"Understanding the 4 Types of Strength." 2020. Invictus Fitness. June 13, 2020. Accessed April 5, 2022. https://www.crossfitinvictus.com/blog/4-types-strength/.

UW Health. 2019. "Eating for Peak Athletic Performance | News | UW Health." Www.uwhealth.org. March 4, 2019. https://www.uwhealth.org/news/eating-for-peak-athletic-performance.

"Vitamins." 2019. The Nutrition Source. February 15, 2019. https://www.hsph.harvard.edu/nutritionsource/vitamins/.

Water Science School. 2019. "The Water in You: Water and the Human Body | U.S. Geological Survey." Www.usgs.gov. May 22, 2019. https://www.usgs.gov/special-topics/water-science-school/science/water-you-water-and-human-body.

"Weight Loss Diet Plans." 2021. Mayo Clinic. November 19, 2021. https://www.mayoclinic.org/healthy-lifestyle/weight-loss/basics/diet-plans/hlv-20049483.

West, Helen. 2018. "The 10 Best Foods That Are High in Zinc." Healthline. 2018. https://www.healthline.com/nutrition/best-foods-high-in-zinc.

West, Helen. 2019. "35 Simple Ways to Cut Lots of Calories." Healthline. Healthline Media. April 23, 2019. https://www.healthline.com/nutrition/35-ways-to-cut-calories.

"What Are Compound Exercise | AFA Blog." 2018. Australian Fitness Academy. October 31, 2018. https://www.fitnesseducation.edu.au/blog/education/what-are-compound-exercises.

"What Are Compound Exercises?" 2021. Columbia Association.

March 30, 2021. https://www.columbiaassociation.org/blog/what-are-compound-exercises.

"What Is Mental Fitness? A How-to for Exercising Your Brain." 2021. Www.betterup.com. September 24, 2021. https://www.betterup.com/blog/what-does-it-mean-to-be-mentally-fit.

"Why Sticking to 80% Diet and 20% Exercise Is Your Best Bet for Weight Loss! - Times of India." 2018. The Times of India. March 22, 2018. https://timesofindia.indiatimes.com/life-style/health-fitness/weight-loss/why-sticking-to-80-diet-and-20-exercise-is-your-best-bet-for-weight-loss/articleshow/63414159.cms.

Wikipedia Contributors. 2018. "Fat." Wikipedia. Wikimedia Foundation. November 26, 2018. https://en.wikipedia.org/wiki/Fat.

Wikipedia Contributors. 2018a. "Water." Wikipedia. Wikimedia Foundation. November 27, 2018. https://en.wikipedia.org/wiki/Water.

Wikipedia Contributors. 2019. "Nutrition." Wikipedia. Wikimedia Foundation. March 23, 2019. https://en.wikipedia.org/wiki/Nutrition.

Wikipedia Contributors. 2019a. "Calorie." Wikipedia. Wikimedia Foundation. July 15, 2019. https://en.wikipedia.org/wiki/Calorie.

Wikipedia Contributors. 2019b. "Metabolism." Wikipedia. Wikimedia Foundation. April 28, 2019. https://en.wikipedia.org/wiki/Metabolism.

Wikipedia Contributors. 2019c. "Physical Fitness." Wikipedia. Wikimedia Foundation. February 26, 2019. https://en.wikipedia.org/wiki/Physical_fitness.

Wikipedia Contributors. 2019d. "Protein." Wikipedia. Wikimedia Foundation. March 10, 2019. https://en.wikipedia.org/wiki/Protein.

Wikipedia Contributors. 2019e. "Bodybuilding." Wikipedia.

Wikimedia Foundation. February 27, 2019. https://en.wikipedia.org/wiki/Bodybuilding.

Wikipedia Contributors. 2019f. "Body Mass Index." Wikipedia. Wikimedia Foundation. April 23, 2019. https://en.wikipedia.org/wiki/Body_mass_index.

Wikipedia Contributors. 2019g. "Adipose Tissue." Wikipedia. Wikimedia Foundation. March 20, 2019. https://en.wikipedia.org/wiki/Adipose_tissue.

Yetman, Daniel. 2020. "Endurance vs. Stamina: Differences and Tips to Improve Both." Healthline. June 12, 2020. https://www.healthline.com/health/exercise-fitness/endurance-vs-stamina.

"Your Better Diet: Top 5 Changes to Make." n.d. WebMD. https://www.webmd.com/health-insurance/features/diet-changes.

Zelman, Kathleen M. 2009. "How Many Calories Do You Really Need?" WebMD. WebMD. August 28, 2009. https://www.webmd.com/diet/guide/calories-chart.